This fully illustrated and easy to follow text provides general practitioners with clear guidelines on how to diagnose and manage the many common genitomedical and sexual health problems seen in general practice. The 'symptom oriented' approach provides quick and clear reference, with essential extra information provided for the more important conditions. Useful advice is given on how to take a sexual history and who to refer on to a genitourinary medicine clinic. The volume covers the full range of commonly occurring male and female genitourinary problems, including those sexually acquired and non-sexually acquired, and also includes chapters on genital problems in children, and advice on contraception.

In addition to being an excellent and practical source of information and advice for the busy general practitioner, it will also be of benefit to practice nurses, other health professionals and medical students entering their clinical years.

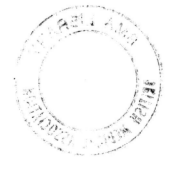

A General Practitioner's Guide to
Genitourinary Medicine and Sexual Health

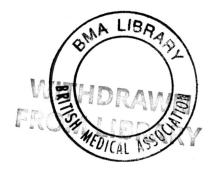

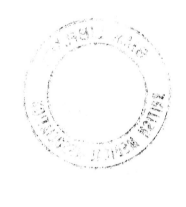

A General Practitioner's Guide to Genitourinary Medicine and Sexual Health

CHRIS SONNEX

Consultant physician in genitourinary medicine, Addenbrooke's Hospital, Cambridge

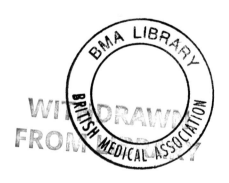

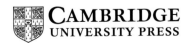

CAMBRIDGE
UNIVERSITY PRESS

Published by the Press Syndicate of the University of Cambridge
The Pitt Building, Trumpington Street, Cambridge CB2 1RP
40 West 20th Street, New York, NY 10011-4211, USA
10 Stamford Road, Oakleigh, Melbourne 3166, Australia

First published 1996

Printed in Great Britain at the University Press, Cambridge

A catalogue record for this book is available from the British Library

Library of Congress cataloguing in publication data

Sonnex, Chris.
A general practitioner's guide to genitourinary medicine and
sexual health/Chris Sonnex.
    p.   cm.
Includes bibliograpical references and index.
ISBN 0 521 55656 2 (hc)
1. Genitourinary organs – Diseases – Handbooks, manuals, etc.   2. Sexually transmitted
diseases – Handbooks, manuals, etc.   3. Physicians (Genital practice) – Handbooks,
manuals, etc.
I. Title.
[DNLM: 1. Genital Diseases, Female.   2. Genital Diseases, Male.   3. Family Practice.
4. Patient Education.   WP 140 S699g 1996]
RC872.9.S65   1996
616.6 – dc20   95–52035 CIP
DNLM/DLC
for Library of Congress

ISBN 0 521 55656 2

VN

CONTENTS

Colour plates may be found facing page 50

FOREWORD

Genitourinary (GU) medicine has been propelled from the backwater of venereology to centre stage in medicine with the advent of diseases like genital herpes, HIV and AIDS. Some of the most sophisticated medical research in the world involves GU medicine and in this heady climate it would be all too easy for GU physicians to forget their colleagues in general practice. Thankfully GU medicine has many bread and butter conditions that it manages well and the 'special clinic' is an important provider of primary medical care. Like general practice the fabric and profile of old style special clinics has improved with up to 25% of clients at a GU medicine clinic attending merely for reassurance: just like in general practice.

General practice is eclectic and is not shy about learning from other disciplines. Most doctors consider themselves non-judgmental but patients do not always consider general practitioners in that light. General practitioners often have difficulties in taking a sexual history, which is understandable as such a history may have to be acquired from people we have known for years in other clinical contexts. It is easier for GU physicians to be dispassionate and clinical about a client's sexual history and probably easier for patients that the doctor seems to have heard it all before. With earlier and increasing sexual activity in adolescence it is likely that general practitioners and GU physicians will have to share each others skills in communications and history taking. A recent study in a large Boston high school showed that 85% of adolescents wanted physicians to given them information on HIV and 67% wished that doctors would ask if they practised safe sex. Seventy per cent of the sample would not be comfortable bringing up sexual matters themselves but are prepared to discuss their sexual anxieties if the topic is broached. The authors concluded that teenagers seemed to view physicians differently from many other adults allowing opportunities for doctors to counsel on sexually related matters (*Paediatrics*, 1995).

While there are aspects of GU medicine that are highly specialised,

GU medicine clinics have retained a strong interest in side room diagnostic procedures. The microscope has largely disappeared from hospital wards and clinics despite its undoubted value. Any general practitioner developing an interest in the GU diseases in his or her practice will find microscopy speeds diagnosis or makes reassurance more compelling. Indeed, 11% of the sample in the 4th National Morbidity Study consulted for genitourinary complaints at least once during the year.

GU medicine and general practice share an interest in educating people about health. Sexual health is of lively interest to doctors, patients and indeed to society. Recent safe sex campaigns have displayed imagination and maturity after the more apocalyptic messages of the mid-1980s. The humble condom continues to play its role in maintaining sexual health and condom usage has increased dramatically. Dr Sonnex gives interesting tips on condom usage which GPs may find invaluable in acquiring 'street cred' with some of their patients.

Most people who suspect they have acquired a sexually transmitted disease will go directly to a GU medicine clinic without recourse to a GP. As GPs we may have to deal with patients who suspect they may have been given a sexually transmitted disease (STD) by someone they know. It is more complex still if the GP suspects a patient has an STD but the patient is apparently unaware of the possibility. This is the stuff of many a GP training session. Innocent parties find it difficult to attend the STD clinic and a host of other issues have to be dealt with by couples who may be in a stable relationship. This commonly involves the GP in negotiating referral to an understanding GU physician and subsequently dealing with the feelings of guilt and/or betrayal felt by the patient. Thus GU infections are unlike almost any other infection in that they cause enormous social and emotional problems. A GU medicine clinic working well with a GP can minimise the trauma for both patient and doctors.

For GPs, and indeed their practice nurses, wishing to respond competently and effectively to the genitourinary complaints of their patients this book will be extremely valuable. As Dr Sonnex demonstrates so well that good clinical practice in GU medicine fits in well with good general practice.

Professor Tom O'Dowd
Department of Community Health
and General Practice
Trinity College
University of Dublin

INTRODUCTION

Genitourinary medicine or GU medicine is a relatively new medical speciality which has developed from the rather more traditional and restricted field of venereology. The diagnosis and management of sexually transmitted diseases (STDs) forms an important part of the workload; however, in recent years we have begun to appreciate that the expertise of GU medicine extends beyond that of pure venereology. A large number of patients now quite appropriately attend our clinics with a variety of non-sexually acquired conditions. The stigma associated with the old-style 'VD Clinic' or 'Special Clinic' unfortunately still lingers and hence many patients may be deterred from attending. The change of name to 'Department of Genitourinary Medicine' or 'GU Medicine Clinic' is leading, albeit slowly, to an improved image and many people (lay and medically qualified) now appreciate that having a sexually transmitted infection is not a prerequisite for clinic attendance. Many clinics provide a colposcopy service and some will have treatment facilities such as laser, cold coagulation or LLETZ, available on site. In addition, a number of clinics now provide regular sessions for family planning and psychosexual medicine.

Most women with an abnormal vaginal discharge present initially to their general practitioner for advice, but referral of the more difficult or persistent cases to GU medicine would now be considered an appropriate next step in management. As microscopy is performed on site a diagnosis can often be made within a few minutes; this is particularly true for the two commonest causes of vaginal discharge: candidiasis and bacterial vaginosis. The ability to undertake microscopy of genital secretions together with the extremely close link with the microbiology laboratory serves to emphasise the important role played by GU medicine in diagnosing genital infection, whether it be sexually or non-sexually acquired.

For the patient with a sexually transmitted infection, the GU medicine clinic provides expert guidance and advice on 'contact tracing' or 'partner notification'. This is an essential part of STD control that requires time and a skilful approach, particularly in cases where the patient does not wish to approach a sexual partner directly. As with most out-patient departments, the range of facilities available and the atmosphere or ambience generated will vary from clinic to clinic. Some will certainly have more of a 'well woman' or 'sexual health clinic' feel to them, others may still carry over traces of the 'VD Clinic' image, although fortunately such clinics are now uncommon.

The objective of this book is to provide the general practitioner with an overview of the type of conditions that could be referred to a department of GU medicine and suggest ways in which genital problems can be best approached and managed. Practice nurses will also hopefully find certain chapters helpful and informative.

I have attempted to make the case for wider referral, which includes those patients with non-STD genital problems, but the primary objective of GU medicine should not be forgotten: that is to control the spread of STDs within the community. Some of my colleagues will rightly argue that we should be striving for a wider brief, that is to improve 'sexual health'. This, together with an emphasis towards destigmatising STDs, should be our ultimate goals. Achieving the right balance between maintaining anonymity and confidentiality for patients with STDs and at the same time providing a more open, general out-patient clinic approach for the patient with, for example, genital dermatitis or recurrent candidiasis can prove very difficult and remains one of the major challenges for the speciality. Only through public education and by close liaison, cross re-ferral and open discussion with our colleagues in general practice and allied specialities such as dermatology, gynaecology and urology will this balance be truly achieved.

ACKNOWLEDGEMENTS

A special thanks to my friend and colleague Chris Carne for his comments and encouragement. I am also indebted to the following for their invaluable input to the various chapters: Pauline Cooper, Andrew Doble, Anthea Edgar, Sarah Edwards, Mark Farrington, Lynne Gilbert, Alan Gelson, Elaine Haigh, Peter Hollis, Helen Hutchinson, Jane MacDougall, Sarah Rann, Steve Tavare, Catherina Thomas, Pat Tate, David Vickers, Martyn Williams and Tim Wreghitt.

CHAPTER 1

Which patients to refer to genitourinary medicine

There is an appreciable overlap between genitourinary medicine and gynae-cology, urology and dermatology which sometimes leads to difficulties when deciding to whom to turn for further advice or a specialist opinion. The following should be considered as general guidelines: if in doubt whether to refer give your local GU medicine clinic a call.

Consider urgent referral

Men with
- urethral discharge or dysuria
- acute epididymitis.

Men and women with
- primary genital herpes
- genital ulceration: previously unconfirmed diagnosis.

Referral strongly recommended

Men and women with:
- Concern (patient or doctor) regarding sexually transmitted infection
- Concern regarding human immunodeficiency virus (HIV) infection
- Any of the following infections:
  - *Chlamydia*
  - non-gonococcal urethritis
  - gonorrhoea
  - genital warts
  - trichomoniasis.
- Sexual partners of patients with:
  - *Chlamydia*

- non-gonococcal urethritis
- gonorrhoea
- genital warts
- trichomoniasis.
- Positive syphilis serology.

Referral recommended

Women with:
- persistent/recurrent vaginal discharge
- chronic pelvic pain
- dysuria/frequency with sterile urine culture
- persistent/recurrent vulval irritation/soreness/burning
- inflammatory cervical cytology (particularly in young, single women using non-barrier contraception or in women with more than one inflammatory smear).

Men with:
- 'testicular'/intrascrotal discomfort
- symptoms suggestive of prostatitis
- balanoposthitis.

Men and women with:
- genital warts
- genital 'lumps' of uncertain aetiology
- genital molluscum contagiosum
- pubic lice
- genital rashes (diagnosis uncertain or unresponsive to treatment).

Consider referral

Women with recurrent candidiasis or recurrent bacterial vaginosis.

Many consultants in GU medicine have specific interests and the services available from individual clinics may vary accordingly. A large number of clinics now provide expertise in vulval disease, psychosexual medicine, colposcopy and rape victim assessment and management. Getting to know your local department of GU medicine or sexual health is to be strongly recommended: most GU medicine clinicians are very approachable and are delighted to have GPs and practice nurses attend clinical sessions and learn more about the speciality.

CHAPTER 2

Routine investigations performed in genitourinary medicine

Patients attending GU medicine for the first time and those with new problems will usually undergo a variety of investigations to check for evidence of infection, both sexually and non-sexually acquired. Many GPs are uncertain which tests are routinely performed and a standard letter from the clinic stating that 'the screen for genital infection proved negative' is not particularly instructive. All clinics should be screening for the same infections; however, the specific tests used may vary from clinic to clinic.

Tests routinely performed are as follows:
(An asterisk indicates tests that may not be currently available or performed in all clinics; polymorphs, polymorphonuclear leucocytes or 'pus cells'; ELISA, enzyme-linked immunosorbent assay.)

Men

URETHRAL SWAB

Gram stain – microscopy
  - >4 polymorphs per high power field (HPF) = urethritis
  - Gram-negative diplococci within polymorphs
    presumptive diagnosis of gonococcal urethritis
Culture for *Neisseria gonorrhoeae*.

*URETHRAL SWAB

Chlamydia trachomatis detection (usually by ELISA or microimmunofluorescence).

TWO GLASS URINE TEST

First glass = a first catch urine (50 ml)
Second glass = second part of urinary stream (50 ml)
Any remaining urine is passed into the urinal.

Interpretation of urine results:

(1) First: clear; second: clear
    = normal
(2) First: pus (seen as threads, flakes, general haze)
    Second: clear
        = anterior urethritis (e.g. NGU (non-gonococcal urethritis), gonorrhoea)
(3) First: pus
    Second: pus
        = posterior urethritis or cystitis (e.g. *E. coli*, etc.)
    Send the first glass urine or a mid-stream urine (MSU) for culture.

Phosphaturia is a common cause of cloudy urine. The addition of acetic acid will clear the urine when excess phosphates are present whereas the haze remains in cases of pyuria.

The urine will also be routinely checked by dipstix.

The details for women are summarised in Table 2.1.

Men and women

SYPHILIS SEROLOGY

A blood sample is routinely taken for syphilis serology. The commonly used tests are the VDRL and TPHA. Screening in ante-natal clinics, GU medicine and on donating blood for transfusion has proved successful in keeping syphilis prevalence extremely low in the U.K.

HEPATITIS SCREENING

Many clinics offer hepatitis B screening and vaccination for injecting drug users and homosexual men and hepatitis C screening for injecting drug users.

HIV ANTIBODY TESTING

Not yet routinely performed without consent. The issue of HIV antibody

Table 2.1. *Routine tests performed on women*

Procedure	Test	Diagnosis
Vaginal swab	Gram stain: microscopy	Assess bacterial flora Bacterial vaginosis Candidiasis
	Wet mount: microscopy	Trichomoniasis Candidiasis
	Culture	*Candida* **Trichomonas vaginalis*
Cervical swab	Gram stain: microscopy	$>$ 30 polymorphs/HPF suggests cervicitis Gram-negative diplococci inside polymorphs → presumptive diagnosis of gonorrhoea
	Culture	*Neisseria gonorrhoeae*
Cervical swab	*Chlamydia trachomatis* detection	
Cervical cytology	(if considered appropriate)	
Urethral swab	Gram stain: microscopy	Polymorphs may be seen in: chlamydial infection gonorrhoea trichomoniasis. Gram-negative diplococci inside polymorphs → presumptive diagnosis of gonorrhoea
	Culture	*Neisseria gonorrhoeae*
*Urethral swab	*Chlamydia trachomatis* detection	

testing is often raised during the consultation and many patients proceed to have a test after the appropriate discussion (Chapter 20). Some clinics provide a 'fast testing service' where results are available the next day. This aims to encourage individuals to be tested who are otherwise deterred by the prospect of a wait for several days for the results.

CHAPTER 3

Taking a sexual history

Whereas most patients attending GU medicine will expect to be asked questions about sex, this is by no means always the case in general practice, even though the patient may have presented with genital symptoms. GU medicine clinicians spend their days asking patients fairly intimate questions about sexual habits and lifestyle and therefore feel comfortable with the questions and the replies. Most GPs will only infrequently need to take a sexual history and a degree of uncertainty regarding which questions to ask and how best to ask them is inevitable. The purpose of this short chapter is to provide basic guidelines on how to approach the patient presenting with genital symptoms or who is concerned that they may have acquired an infection from a sexual partner.

An unmarried female patient presenting with vaginal discharge provides a useful example of one possible approach to sexual history taking.

Important questions are:
- How long has the discharge been present?
- Is there any malodour? (? bacterial vaginosis)
- Is there any associated vulval irritation or soreness? (? candidiasis)
- Have there ever been any previous similar episodes?
  If so:
  - what was the diagnosis?
  - which treatments have been used?
  - have any previous treatments helped?
- Have you experienced any pelvic pain? (? endometritis/pelvic inflammatory disease (PID))
- Has there been any bleeding between periods? (? endometritis)
- When was your last period?
- Has there been any discomfort or pain during sexual intercourse (the terms 'when making love' or 'when having sex' are preferred by some clinicians; use whichever you think will be appropriate for the patient and with which you feel comfortable)

— When did you last have intercourse/have sex/make love?
— Was this your regular partner?
  (1) If no:
    — was this with someone you know well or a fairly casual contact?
    — was this a male partner or a female partner?
    — was he or she from this country?
    — had they recently spent any time abroad?
    — have you had sex with any other partners in the past few months?
  (2) If yes:
    — is this a male partner or a female partner?
    — when did you last have sexual contact with someone other than your regular partner? (This may be more appropriate left to the end of the consultation.)

> Direct eye to eye contact usually works best for the more intimate questions. The last question can be difficult as patients are usually embarrassed to admit an 'extramarital' or casual affair, so you need to try to achieve a lack of surprise and concern whatever the reply.

    — If a male partner: has he mentioned that he has symptoms? For example, a penile rash or any discomfort passing urine?
    — What are you using for contraception? (Consistent use of condoms provides good protection against *Chlamydia* and gonorrhoea)
    — Are you currently on any medication? (Some antibiotics predispose to candidiasis. Fixed drug eruptions may present as fairly extensive areas of erythema or ulceration on the external genitalia.)

You will appreciate that a number of these questions are aimed specifically at determining the risk of sexually transmitted infection. They may not be relevant to the patient with clinically obvious vaginal 'thrush' but should be considered in women with, for example, troublesome vaginal discharge unresponsive to treatment.

If a woman's last sexual contact was with another woman, it is worth enquiring when they last had sexual contact with a man. Women who are exclusively lesbian are unlikely to have chlamydial or gonococcal infection whereas bacterial vaginosis appears to be slightly more common in lesbian than in heterosexual women.

A similar line of questioning to the above is required for men attending with genital symptoms such as dysuria, urethral discharge, epididymal tenderness or genital ulceration. You should directly enquire:

- when they last had sexual intercourse
- whether this was with a 'regular' or 'casual' partner
- whether this was with a male or female partner
- whether there have been other sexual contacts in the previous few months.

With gay men, one should also obtain a little more detail about clinically relevant sexual practices. For example:

Do you usually practice 'safe-sex'? (e.g. body-rubbing, mutual masturbation)?
When did you last have penetrative intercourse?
When you have penetrative intercourse are you usually 'active' (ano-insertive) or 'passive' (ano-receptive)?
- if predominantly 'active', when were you last 'passive'?
- if predominantly 'passive', when were you last 'active'?
- do you routinely/always use condoms?
- are you having any problems with condoms splitting or tearing? (extra-strong condoms are available, e.g. Durex 'Ultra Strong', Mates 'Super Strong'; certain lubricants can damage condom latex (see also p. 48)
When did you last have oral sex? (Some infections can be passed from the throat to the urethra, e.g. non-specific urethritis (NSU), gonorrhoea. HIV may also be transmitted by orogenital contact)
Were you active and/or receptive? (i.e. your penis into partner's mouth or vice versa).

Other sexual practices that may lead to the transmission of infection or clinical complications include:

- 'rimming' (oro-anal contact): intestinal pathogens, hepatitis A
- 'fisting' (hand insertion into rectum): damage to the anal sphincter, rectal tears.

The issue of HIV infection should be raised if the history suggests a possibility of potentially risky sexual practices. Recent studies suggest that a number of young homosexual men perceive HIV as a problem affecting the 'older generation' and are reverting to unsafe sexual practices, in particular, unprotected anal intercourse with casual partners.

CHAPTER 4

Bacterial vaginosis

Bacterial vaginosis (BV) is more common than 'thrush' and is probably the commonest cause of abnormal vaginal discharge seen in general practice. The condition is certainly underdiagnosed and frequently misdiagnosed. BV was formerly known as 'Gardnerella' and is caused by an overgrowth of predominantly anaerobic bacterial species which are commonly present in low concentrations in the healthy vagina (e.g. *Gardnerella vaginalis*, *Bacteroides* spp., *Peptostreptococcus*, *Mobiluncus*, *Mycoplasma hominis*).

Although many clinicians regard BV as a fairly insignificant condition this is certainly not the case for the majority of sufferers. Many women find the amount of discharge, and in some cases the associated malodour, to be particularly distressing. In addition, there is increasing evidence that BV is associated with preterm labour, chorioamnionitis, postpartum endometritis and bacteraemia, pelvic infection following surgery and termination of pregnancy and, possibly, PID.

Symptoms

The commonest presenting symptom is excessive vaginal discharge, sometimes with a slight malodour. Some women regard a fishy vaginal odour as normal and are surprised and grateful when BV is eventually diagnosed and treated. Malodour may only be noticeable after unprotected sexual intercourse, owing to the release of amines by alkaline semen (see 'amine test' below). Vulval irritation is uncommon. As with candidiasis, many women with BV are asymptomatic.

Diagnosis

The two most important methods of diagnosis are:

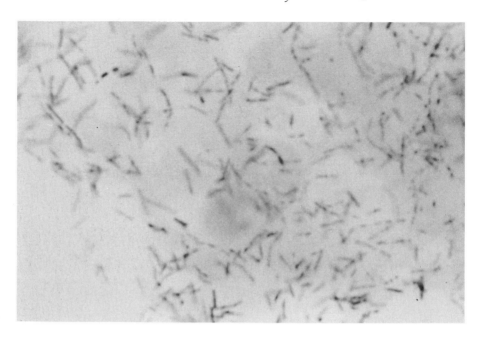

Fig. 4.1 Gram stain appearance of normal vaginal secretions showing predominance of lactobacilli.

(1) Microscopy of vaginal secretions
    BV produces a highly characteristic appearance on Gram staining. There is an absence of lactobacilli and an excess of Gram-variable or Gram-negative rods (*Gardnerella, Bacteroides, Peptostreptococcus*; Figs 4.1 and 4.2). In some cases Gram-negative 'curved rods' (*Mobiluncus*) may be seen. As vaginal inflammation (vaginitis) is not a feature of BV, few polymorphs are present.

(2) Amine test
    This test involves the addition of two drops of 1–5% potassium hydroxide solution to a sample of the vaginal secretions, either on a slide or swab. The sudden release of a fishy odour represents a 'positive' result. The odour results from volatilisation of polyamines, in particular trimethylamine, that are thought to be produced by the anaerobic bacteria.
    Compared with microscopy, the 'amine test' has a sensitivity of 80–90% and a specificity of well over 90%. The test is easy, quick and inexpensive to perform and should be part of the initial assessment of all women with vaginal discharge.
    Although the amine test may be performed on air-dried swabs some hours or days later, the main advantage of the test is that it can be

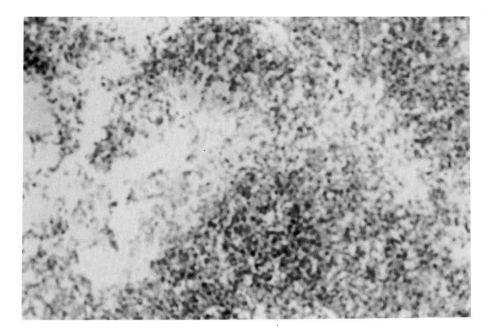

Fig. 4.2 Bacterial vaginosis. Typical Gram stain appearance. Loss of lactobacilli with other organisms (e.g. *Gardnerella vaginalis*, *Bacteroides* spp.) predominating.

performed during the consultation. The odour produced is short lasting and, despite some claims to the contrary, does not linger in the room where the test is performed. Testing should ideally take place out of sight of the patient.

Other diagnostic criteria mentioned in the textbooks but less helpful than microscopy and amine testing are:

(3) Vaginal pH

In BV, vaginal pH is raised from the normal value of 4.5 to above 5.0. Unfortunately, this is not specific and probably signifies simply a reduction in the number of lactobacilli. In addition, a raised pH may be found in a woman with a normal vaginal flora if testing is performed when menstrual blood or semen is present or if cervical mucus is inadvertently sampled instead of vaginal secretions. BV, however, is very unlikely to be present if the pH is normal.

(4) Appearance of the discharge

Although the vaginal discharge in BV is classically thin, homogeneous with a creamy or milky consistency and a slight froth (Fig. 4.3), this is by no means always the case, and in most studies the appearance of vaginal fluid has been shown to be a poor diagnostic marker.

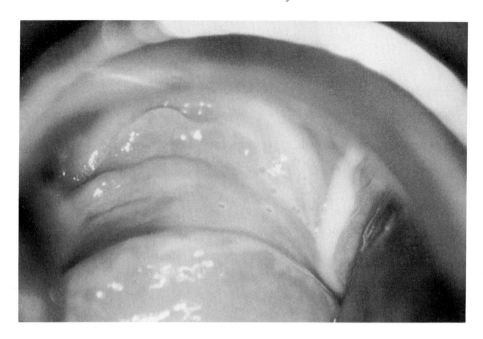

Fig. 4.3 Bacterial vaginosis. Homogeneous discharge coating vaginal wall.

High vaginal swab culture has no place in diagnosis because the presence of *Gardnerella vaginalis* or anaerobes does not necessarily indicate the presence of bacterial vaginosis. Quantitative culture may be helpful but is difficult to perform. As mentioned above, microscopy is the diagnostic test of choice.

Treatment

Treatment is currently reserved for women with symptoms. A case could be made for treating asymptomatic women prior to hysterectomy, endometrial biopsy, dilatation and curettage (D & C), intrauterine contraceptive device (IUCD) insertion and termination of pregnancy. Trials are ongoing to assess whether treatment in pregnancy reduces the risk of preterm labour. On current evidence, treatment should be considered in pregnant women with previous preterm labour or late miscarriage.

– Oral metronidazole is an extremely effective treatment and various regimens have been used: 2 g suspension stat dose; 400–800 mg bd for 2 days; 200 mg tds for 7 days.

- Intravaginal 2% clindamycin cream is a useful alternative for patients who cannot tolerate metronidazole.
- Ampicillin 500 mg qds for 7 days or ciproflaxacin 250 mg bd for 7 days have been used in some cases but appear to be less effective than metronidazole or clindamycin.

Recurrent bacterial vaginosis

Treating sexual partners has been shown to have NO effect on reducing the recurrence rate. There is an association between BV and the IUCD. In women with particularly troublesome recurrences an alternative form of contraception should be considered. Using condoms for a few months may prove beneficial for some patients. A short course of oral metronidazole or intravaginal clindamycin once or twice a month may also be worth considering as a prophylactic measure (the necessary studies are awaited).

CHAPTER 5

Candidiasis

General practitioners are all too familiar with this condition, so there is little to be gained by reiterating common knowledge. There are, however, a few points worth making.

Although *Candida albicans* is the commonest cause of vulvovaginal infection, other strains such as *Candida tropicalis* and *Candida* (formerly *Torulopsis*) *glabrata*, may also occasionally produce symptoms. *Candida glabrata* is thought to account for about 5% of vaginal infections.

Accurate identification of *Candida* spp. is particularly important when dealing with persistent or recurrent infection; however, this identification may not be available routinely in all microbiology laboratories. Non-*albicans* strains of *Candida* often show partial or complete resistance to the commonly used topical and oral antifungal agents.

Oral antifungals (e.g. fluconazole, itraconazole) are extremely effective, easy to use and appear to be safe. They are, however, rather more expensive than topical treatments and should not be used in pregnancy.

Recurrent candidiasis

A small number of women are plagued by frequent recurrences of vulvovaginal candidiasis. The reasons are unclear, although there is some evidence to suggest a localised *Candida*-specific defect in cell-mediated immunity. When a patient presents complaining of 'recurrent thrush' one of the most important first steps in management is to make sure that the diagnosis is correct.

PRACTICAL POINTS

Whenever possible try to send a vaginal swab for *Candida* culture on each occasion that symptoms are present. Failure to culture the yeast makes the diagnosis less likely.

If symptoms persist and *Candida* continues to be isolated after treatment ask the laboratory to identify the *Candida* sp. and report on its sensitivities to the various antifungals. This will usually require the sample being sent to a reference laboratory. Non-*albicans* strains of *Candida* are often resistant to imidazoles (e.g. clotrimazole, miconazole, econazole) and triazoles (fluconazole, itraconazole) but they may respond to topical nystatin (a polyene).

Consider a trial of an oral antifungal, such as fluconazole 150 mg stat followed by 50 mg daily for 1 week or itraconazole 200 mg bd for 1 day followed by 200 mg daily for 1 week. Lack of clinical response suggests that *Candida* is not the cause of the symptoms or that a resistant strain of *Candida* is present. Symptoms of vulval irritation, with or without discharge, which initially improve with antifungal treatment but then recur some days or weeks later are highly suggestive of candidiasis.

DIFFERENTIAL DIAGNOSES

Consider bacterial vaginosis in a woman with recurrent vaginal discharge that fails to respond to antifungal treatment. Vulval irritation is unusual in this condition.

Vulval dermatoses (see also Chapter 8 on Vulval problems). Seborrhoeic dermatitis, contact dermatitis, psoriasis and lichen sclerosus et atrophicus are just a few of the skin conditions that may present with vulval irritation. Their appearance on the vulva is often atypical and sometimes a biopsy will be required to make the correct diagnosis. In cases of contact dermatitis there is often a history of allergy or a family history of atopy. Potential vulval sensitising agents include topical medications (e.g. Tri-adcortyl, antifungal creams), KY jelly (propylene glycol sensitivity), spermicidal creams, sanitary pads, dyed lavatory paper, bubble-baths and scented soaps.

MANAGEMENT OF RECURRENT CANDIDIASIS

Once you are satisfied that the diagnosis is correct the following points are worth considering.

Screen for other genital infections

Some clinicians believe that *Candida* acts as an opportunistic pathogen in the vagina and that recurrent episodes indicate some other underlying infection. There is only indirect evidence, however, supporting this claim, which comes from a study reporting a higher prevalence of non-specific urethritis (NSU) amongst the male partners of women with recurrent thrush compared with a control group.

Prophylactic antifungals

Women with perimenstrual thrush may benefit from prophylactic antifungal therapy either before or just after the period. This can be as a single clotrimazole 500 mg pessary or fenticonazole 600 mg pessary, oral fluconazole 150 mg or itraconazole 200 mg bd for 1 day. Some women will require fortnightly treatment and very occasionally weekly prophylaxis. This regimen should be continued for 3–6 months, then stopped and the situation reassessed.

Treatment of male sexual partners

Treating the male partner with an antifungal cream does not reduce the frequency of recurrent episodes in the female. Men should therefore only receive treatment if they have evidence of candidal infection themselves. As mentioned above, it may be worth screening male partners for asymptomatic NSU. This may lead to infection in the female, which may be difficult to detect on routine investigation, and predispose to recurrent attacks of thrush.

Treatment of the 'gut reservoir'

Early studies suggested that recurrences of vaginal candidiasis result from reinfection from the gut. This is now considered unlikely and indeed more recent work has failed to show any benefit from the use of oral nystatin. Intestinal colonisation with *Candida* therefore appears to play no role in recurrent vaginal infection and can be ignored.

'Deep-seated' vaginal infection

Failure to eradicate *Candida* from the 'deeper layers' of the vaginal mucosa has led some clinicians to suggest using longer courses of antifungal treatment. This is still an issue of debate, but consider treating acute recurrences with a 2-week course of antifungal pessaries or oral agents.

Diet

There is no evidence to suggest that a diet high in sugars or carbohydrates predisposes to thrush. One recent study of particular interest has reported a reduction in vaginal *Candida* colonisation among women ingesting 8 ounces of yoghurt daily. A 'natural' yoghurt was used supposedly containing *Lactobacillus acidophilus*. Although this work requires confirmation with a larger number of patients and a placebo arm, yoghurt supplementation sounds attractive and would probably be well accepted. Interestingly, many of the so-called 'live' or 'natural' yoghurt products on the market do not contain *Lactobacillus acidophilus* or contain only 'non-vaginal' strains of lactobacilli. A small number of studies have shown an association between low zinc status and recurrent vaginal infection including recurrent candidiasis. This has led some clinicians to suggest a trial of oral zinc supplements for 1 or 2 months in women with particularly troublesome thrush. Garlic contains an antifungal, allicin, and has been advocated as a treatment for thrush; however, current evidence suggests that the amount of garlic required to provide clinically useful levels of allicin in the vagina may be socially unacceptable. Nevertheless, natural remedies are very fashionable and further study is certainly warranted.

Diabetes

Poorly controlled diabetes may predispose to thrush, but it is very uncommon to find diabetes in women with recurrent infection; however, it is prudent to dipstix the urine.

Oral contraceptive pill

Theoretical evidence suggests that the pill could play a role in potentiating vaginal candidiasis. A cytosol receptor for oestrogen has been reported in *Candida albicans* and certain hormones have been shown *in vitro* to stimulate yeast mycelial formation and hence virulence. In spite of this evidence, recent studies have failed to show an association between low-moderate dose oral contraceptive pill use and recurrent candidiasis.

Iron deficiency anaemia

This does not predispose to recurrent thrush.

Bubble-baths and scented soaps

The irritation associated with candidal vulvitis may be aggravated by bubble-baths and scented soaps. Conversely, epithelial damage due to a mild contact dermatitis to one of the chemicals in a bubble-bath or soap may predispose to symptomatic candidiasis.

Tight-fitting clothing

Women with recurrent thrush are often advised to avoid wearing nylon underwear and tights. The theory is that the increased humidity generated by the nylon may lead to mild epithelial maceration and subsequently lead to fungal invasion of the superficial tissue and hence to symptomatic infection. This is anecdotal but loose clothing does provide a degree of comfort to some women.

Antibiotics

A number of women are prone to develop thrush during courses of oral antibiotics. This may be due to the elimination of the protective vaginal lactobacilli or to a direct potentiating effect on yeast growth. Prescribing a course of antifungals along with the antibiotics is worth considering and is usually well appreciated.

Douches

Vinegar douches provide symptomatic relief for some women. It should be remembered that douching may facilitate the spread of lower genital tract bacteria into the uterus and is not to be generally recommended.

Boric acid

Gelatin capsules of boric acid have been successfully used to treat persistent vaginal candidiasis, in particular *Candida glabrata* infection. The recommended dosage is 600 mg bd and as the capsules are not generally available these need to be made up by a kindly pharmacist.

Hormonal therapy

There are anecdotal reports of successful treatments of persistent *Candida glabrata* infection with progestogens, for example dydrogesterone or medroxyprogesterone acetate.

Summary of recurrent/persistent vaginal candidiasis

1. Make sure that the diagnosis is correct.
2. Identify *Candida* spp. and check sensitivities to the antifungals prescribed.
3. Treat initially with a longer course of antifungals.
4. Use monthly or fortnightly oral or topical antifungals for 3–6 months as prophylaxis.
5. No need to treat male partners with antifungals unless symptomatic.
6. Consider screening for other genital infections.

CHAPTER 6

Other causes of vaginal discharge

Trichomoniasis

This has become less common in recent years and usually presents as quite a heavy yellow discharge associated with vulval and vaginal soreness. The motile trichomonads are easily seen on wet-mount microscopy (i.e. examination of a sample of vaginal discharge in a drop of normal saline under a coverslip; Fig. 6.1); however, as this is rarely available in non-GU medicine settings, the diagnosis should be made by vaginal swab culture.

Treatment is with oral metronidazole, preferably a 2 g stat dosage, although 200 mg tds for 7 days may be used. Metronidazole is better tolerated if taken with or after food and alcohol should be avoided during treatment and for 24 h afterwards.

Most cases of trichomoniasis are sexually transmitted; sexual partners should therefore be assessed and treated. Men usually carry the infection without symptoms.

Streptococcal infection

Lancefield Group A and Group B streptococci are uncommon causes of vaginitis. Only approximately 50% of women with Group B infection report symptoms, usually vaginal soreness and irritation. Group A infection is less common but more likely to produce symptoms. There is frequently a marked vaginitis with a serosanguineous discharge.

Foreign objects

Liberal views on sexual experimentation has led to various devices becoming lodged or even lost in the vagina. Although the patient is usually

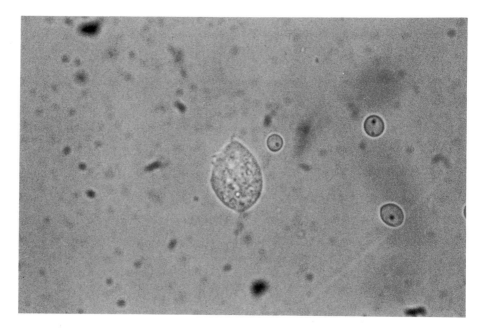

Fig. 6.1 *Trichomonas vaginalis.* Diagnosis by wet-mount microscopy.

only too aware that something has 'gone missing', occasionally bits of 'sex toys' can break off unknowingly and give rise to a vaginal discharge some days later.

More commonly a tampon can inadvertently be pushed deep into the vagina and be forgotten. After a few days this produces an unpleasant smelling discharge. Bits of tampons occasionally latch onto threads of an IUCD and cause later problems. These small pieces of cotton wool can often be very difficult to detect. Similarly, small fragments of toilet paper can be left at the entrance of the vagina following a hurried wipe after urination. Sexual activity can push these deep into the vagina only to produce a discharge after a few days.

Very occasionally condoms split during intercourse with the result that fragments of rubber may be retained in the vagina and eventually give rise to a malodorous discharge.

Cervicitis

Cervical inflammation may cause a mucopurulent discharge which, although originating from the cervix, presents as a vaginal discharge.

IMPORTANT POINTS

1. Cervicitis is often difficult to distinguish from cervical ectopy as in both cases the cervix appears red to the naked eye. Indicators of cervicitis include mucopurulent secretions (Plate 6.1) and contact bleeding on touching the cervix with a cotton wool swab, e.g. when taking an endocervical swab for *Chlamydia* (not when scraping the cervix with a wooden spatula for cervical cytology). In GU medicine, cervical secretions are examined under the microscope and the number of polymorphs present quantified. A count of greater than 30 polymorphs per HPF is highly suggestive of a cervicitis.

   A cervical ectopy may produce excessive mucus in the absence of infection. This can be treated by cryotherapy or diathermy but should only be considered when infection has been adequately checked for and discounted.

2. *Chlamydia trachomatis* is the commonest cause of cervicitis in the U.K. Remember to gently wipe the cervix clear of discharge before taking a swab for *Chlamydia*. Cellular material rather than mucus is required for diagnosis.

3. Although gonorrhoea is less common than *Chlamydia*, a swab should be taken from the cervix for *Neisseria gonorrhoeae* culture. The gonococcus is a fragile organism and therefore the sample must be transported to the laboratory as soon as possible; if there is likely to be an overnight delay then keep the swab at room temperature rather than in the refrigerator. Women with suspected gonorrhoea should ideally be referred to GU medicine. The appropriate swabs from the cervix (not vagina), urethra, rectum and pharynx can then be taken and plated directly on to specific media and incubated prior to transport to the laboratory. Owing to the anatomical close proximity of anus and vagina, rectal infection may be present in the absence of a history of anal intercourse.

4. In many cases no causative organism can be found and the diagnosis is one of 'non-specific cervicitis' (the female equivalent of 'non-specific urethritis').

MANAGEMENT OF CERVICITIS

Non-specific cervicitis and chlamydial infection should be treated with a tetracycline (e.g. doxycycline 100 mg bd for 10–14 days), erythromycin (a 14-day course is usually required to treat adequately a chlamydial infection) or azithromycin 1 g stat. Sexual partners should be assessed for urethritis; this is often asymptomatic. Failure to treat partners may lead to reinfection.

As mentioned above, patients with suspected gonorrhoea should be referred to GU medicine for treatment, follow-up and contact tracing. If the diagnosis of gonorrhoea has been confirmed by culture and there is a delay before the patient can be seen by GU medicine, consider treating with oral ampicillin 2 g stat plus probenecid 1 g stat and then refer to GU medicine for follow-up and contact tracing.

Penicillin-resistant gonorrhoea is seen in the U.K., mostly in patients who have had sexual contact with partners from outside the U.K. Ciprofloxacin 500 mg stat is currently the recommended treatment for penicillin-resistant cases, although strains resistant to 4-quinolones are occasionally seen in the U.K. Most laboratories will provide details of antibiotic sensitivities for their gonococcal isolates.

Prescribing a 10-day course of tetracycline in addition to antigonococcal treatment to cover possible co-infection with *Chlamydia* is to be recommended.

Physiological discharge

Many women present with excessive vaginal discharge for which no infective cause can be found. In some cases this will be an increased awareness or a true increase in volume of normal vaginal secretions. Desquamated vaginal epithelial cells, cervical mucus and transudated fluid from the vaginal mucosa are the main constituents of normal vaginal secretions and the amount produced may vary with the phase of the menstrual cycle. It is worth emphasising that physiological discharge should only be diagnosed when both microscopy and culture of vaginal and cervical secretions prove negative; a clinical judgement is insufficient. Explaining the nature of the discharge and providing reassurance that no infection is present is often all that is required in the way of management. If the discharge is particularly troublesome, gentle douching with a povidone-iodine solution may be considered; because of the increased risk of pelvic infection associated with douching it is important to ensure that infection is absent, in particular bacterial vaginosis and *Chlamydia*.

Some women with cervical ectopy produce an excessive amount of mucus and will often describe their discharge as 'thick and stringy'. Non-infected cervical mucus is clear; white or yellow mucus is highly suggestive of infection. Irrespective of the clinical findings the appropriate swabs must be taken to check for infection (see above) in addition to cervical cytology, if this has not been performed recently. Treatment with cryotherapy or diathermy should be considered once infection and cervical pathology have been excluded.

CHAPTER 7

A general approach to the management of vaginal discharge

It would be impractical, and indeed unnecessary, to refer all women with an abnormal vaginal discharge to GU medicine. Many women self-diagnose 'thrush' and approach their GP requesting a repeat prescription of anti-fungals without investigation or examination. This is not an ideal approach to management. Confirmatory vaginal swabs should be taken on at least some occasions and if this is considered 'difficult', for whatever reasons, then a GU medicine referral is advisable. There is also some concern that the availability of topical anti-'thrush' treatments without prescription may considerably delay some women from seeking professional help.

There are a few other points worth considering when deciding whether to refer a patient to GU medicine.

1. In addition to obtaining optimal specimens for culture, microscopy of vaginal, cervical and urethral secretions is performed routinely in all GU medicine clinics which enables the clinician to make, in many cases, an immediate diagnosis. Microscopy is an invaluable method of assessing the general health of the vagina and cervix. For example, a woman with symptomatic discharge showing a predominance of lactobacilli on the vaginal Gram stain, a normal cervical Gram stain and negative vaginal and cervical cultures is most likely to have a physiological discharge.
2. The two commonest causes of vaginal discharge seen in general practice and among attenders at GU medicine are candidiasis and bacterial vaginosis, neither of which are sexually transmitted. Microscopy of vaginal secretions is essential to accurately diagnose bacterial vaginosis; high vaginal swab culture is of no use.
3. There are a few key questions that may give a clue to the diagnosis:
   – Irritation or soreness is suggestive of candidiasis.
   – A malodorous discharge is suggestive of bacterial vaginosis.

— Intermenstrual bleeding or pelvic discomfort, a recent change of sexual partner and the use of non-barrier contraception increase the likelihood of sexually transmitted infection.

4. Which swabs to take. A Stuart's swab for microbiological culture is usually adequate to detect genital tract pathogens. It is important that the swab reaches the laboratory as soon as possible: *Trichomonas vaginalis* and the gonococcus are particularly delicate and may not survive an overnight delay before reaching specific culture media.

Keep genital specimens at room temperature rather than in the refrigerator if there is likely to be a delay before reaching the laboratory.

If gonorrhoea is considered a possible diagnosis the patient should be referred to GU medicine so that the appropriate swabs may be taken (i.e. urethral, cervical, rectal and pharyngeal but NOT vaginal), plated on to the appropriate culture media and incubated prior to transport to the laboratory.

Chlamydia trachomatis is usually diagnosed by antigen detection methods, such as ELISA or microimmunofluorescence. Wipe the cervix clear of vaginal secretions before taking an endocervical sample (i.e. a sample from the columnar epithelium) and remember that cellular material rather than mucus is required for diagnosis. A 1–2 day delay in transport should not adversely affect the results. It is worth emphasising that even with a perfectly taken clinical specimen the currently available tests for *Chlamydia* may yield false positive or false negative results. Many laboratories will routinely retest positive samples using a different antigen detection method from the original test. A positive result on both tests is likely to indicate a true infection. The significance of equivocal results must be judged on clinical merit.

Bacterial vaginosis cannot be diagnosed from a vaginal swab unless a Gram stain is prepared.

Guidelines for the management of vaginal discharge are summarised in Table 7.1.

Table 7.1. *Diagnosis and management of vaginal discharge*

	Diagnosis
1. Take a history	
Any suggestion of sexually transmitted infection (e.g. recent change of sexual partner)	
Vulval irritation or soreness	Candidiasis or trichomoniasis
Malodour	Bacterial vaginosis
2. Examination	
Vulval/vaginal erythema	Candidiasis or trichomoniasis
'Lumpy' or 'curd-like' discharge	Candidiasis
Smooth, homogeneous, slightly frothy discharge	Bacterial vaginosis
Moderately heavy yellow discharge	Trichomoniasis; cervicitis
Yellow cervical mucus ± contact bleeding on gently swabbing the cervix	Cervicitis
3. Investigations	
(a) Vaginal swab (e.g. Stuart's) (Probably not worth taking if > 24 h delay before arriving in laboratory) (Keep specimen at room temperature – NOT in refrigerator)	Candidiasis, trichomoniasis, Streptococcal infection
(b) Second vaginal swab Roll gently onto microscope slide AIR dry Ask laboratory to Gram stain	Bacterial vaginosis
Before discarding, drop 1–5% KOH onto swab and sniff → pronounced 'fish-like' odour = positive 'amine' test	Bacterial vaginosis
If sexually transmitted infection a possibility or clinical suspicion of cervicitis → refer to GU medicine clinic If patient unwilling or impractical to attend:	
(a) Cervical swab: Stuart's (send to laboratory as soon as possible)	Gonorrhoea

Table 7.1. (*cont.*)

	Diagnosis
(b) Second cervical swab (special test kits available which contain appropriate swab and transport medium) Also consider taking urethral swabs for *Chlamydia* and gonorrhoea in conjunction with cervical specimens (see text)	*Chlamydia*

4. Management

Diagnosis	Treatment
Candidiasis	A topical imidazole (pessaries and cream), oral fluconazole 150 mg stat, oral itraconazole 200 mg bd for 1 day
Bacterial vaginosis	Oral metronidazole, e.g. 2 g suspension stat 200 mg tds for 7 days 400 mg bd for 2 days Intravaginal 2% clindamycin cream for 7 days
Trichomoniasis	Oral metronidazole, e.g. 2 g suspension stat Sexual partners should be assessed and treated
Chlamydia	Tetracyclines (e.g. doxycycline 100 mg bd for 10 days) Erythromycin (500 mg bd for 14 days) Azithromycin 1 g stat Strongly consider referral to GU medicine for follow-up and contact tracing
Gonorrhoea	Ampicillin 2 g orally stat + probenecid 1 g orally stat Ciprofloxacin 500 mg stat Patients found to have gonorrhoea should be referred to GU medicine for follow-up and contact tracing

bd, twice daily; tds, three times daily; GU, genitourinary; stat, once only.

CHAPTER 8

Vulval problems

Vulval disease is common and although most of the conditions presenting in general practice are straightforward a significant number of women pose rather more of a diagnostic and management problem.

Important points to consider are:

1. What are the predominant symptoms: irritation, soreness or burning?
   Is there an urge to scratch or is the skin too sore?
   Is the whole vulva affected or are symptoms localised to one particular area?
2. Is there a personal or family history of allergy?
3. Any history of skin problems, e.g. dermatitis/eczema, psoriasis, lichen planus?
4. Which soap is used for cleansing the genital area? Are bubble-bath, hygiene sprays, etc. used?
5. Are symptoms related to the time in the menstrual cycle or brought on by coitus?

Although candidiasis is the commonest cause of vulval irritation, this diagnosis should be reconsidered if vaginal swabs fail to grow the fungus and there is no response to antifungal treatment. If there is doubt, consider using a longer course of an oral antifungal (e.g. itraconazole or fluconazole) as a diagnostic test. If there is no clinical response to antifungals in spite of *Candida* being isolated on culture, ask the laboratory to identify the *Candida* spp., as some of the more unusual strains (e.g. *Candida* (*Torulopsis*) *glabrata*) are resistant to the commonly used imidazole preparations.

Although the vulva may be affected by a variety of skin conditions the clinical features are often modified by secondary infection, scratching (causing lichenification or skin thickening) or by previous treatments. Examination of the scalp, nails, elbows and mouth may provide useful clues to the diagnosis.

Vulval irritation

Conditions that may present with vulval irritation include:

1. Candidiasis
   See above, Chapter 5 and Plate 6.2.
2. Human papillomavirus (HPV) infection (see also Chapter 18, p. 77).
   Genital warts can cause slight irritation and when they first appear
   may be quite difficult to identify without some form of magnification,
   such as a colposcope. (Note: Anal warts may present as pruritis ani;
   beware the diagnosis of haemorrhoids without careful examination!)
   Vulval intraepithelial neoplasia (VIN) is strongly associated with HPV
   type 16 infection and often presents as white or off-white, flat or papular
   lesions, most commonly affecting the labia minora and perineum.
   Lesions are multifocal in 70% of women and cause irritation in just
   under two-thirds. Biopsy should be considered to confirm the diagnosis
   and stage the lesion (VIN I, VIN II or VIN III). VIN has the potential to
   progress to invasive carcinoma, particularly in the more mature
   woman, and therefore careful follow-up is advisable. In addition, as
   VIN is associated with dysplasia elsewhere in the genital tract it is
   important to ensure that cervical cytology, and if possible colposcopy,
   is performed on a regular basis, ideally annually.
3. Genital herpes (see also Chapter 17, p. 67).
   Some women report vulval irritation before ulcers appear. With primary genital herpes, the irritation is soon superseded by increasing
   soreness and subsequently ulceration and vulval oedema. The typical
   blisters are fragile and often missed. A history of a 'flu-like' illness or
   sore throat prior to the onset of the vulval symptoms is often a helpful
   diagnostic clue.
      In recurrent herpes, the vulval lesions may be tiny and easily over-
   looked unless the patient or examining clinician is alert to the possible
   diagnosis. Examination with a magnifying glass or colposcope can be
   helpful in these cases.
4. Trichomoniasis
   Trichomonas vaginalis usually causes a vulvovaginitis associated with an
   increased vaginal discharge. Diagnosis is by wet-mount microscopy or
   culture (see p. 19).
5. Streptococcal infection
   Although both Lancefield Group A and Group B streptococci may cause
   a vulvovaginitis, this is uncommon and vulval infection usually occurs
   secondarily to an already damaged vulval skin, e.g. from dermatitis.

Vulval erysipelas is usually associated with Group A streptococci and presents as pronounced labial swelling and erythema which may progress to necrosis.

6. Dermatoses

   These are not uncommon and often involve the labia majora and perineum.

   (a) Seborrhoeic dermatitis (Plate 6.3). Look for evidence elsewhere, such as on the face, chest and scalp.

   (b) Contact dermatitis. There is often a history of allergies or family history of atopy. Check whether any creams or lotions are being applied to the genital area. Latex allergy usually presents as vaginal soreness after using condoms. Seminal fluid, KY jelly or spermicide allergy presents as postcoital vaginal discomfort sometimes associated with vulval oedema. Scented soaps, bubble-baths, hygiene sprays, antimicrobial creams and anaesthetic haemorrhoid creams are potential sensitisers.

   (c) Lichen simplex. Some degree of skin thickening or lichenification is common after chronic scratching. Treatment with a moderately potent topical steroid is often required.

   (d) Lichen planus. Look for evidence elsewhere, particularly in the mouth. Erosive lichen planus is a variant that may present with severe vulvitis and vaginitis.

   (e) Psoriasis. Look for evidence elsewhere, including nail pitting, and ask about family history. Lesions in the genital area may not appear typical as the scale is often lost leaving a red, glazed epithelium.

   (f) Lichen sclerosus et atrophicus (Plate 6.4). Commonly affects the anogenital region in children and adults. Often presents with irritation and less commonly soreness. Sexual intercourse can be painful either because of friction damaging the fragile vulval skin or secondary to tightening of the vaginal introitus resulting from postinflammatory scarring. In the early stages the skin appears white and slightly thinned sometimes with small, superficial erosions and 'blood blisters'. Untreated, the inflammatory process may lead to resorption of the labia minora and clitoris and narrowing of the introitus. Active disease should be treated initially with a potent topical steroid (e.g. clobetasol propionate). Long-term follow-up is recommended because of the small risk (up to 4%) of developing squamous cell carcinoma.

Vulval soreness or tenderness

All of the above conditions may cause soreness in addition to or rather than irritation.

FOCAL VULVITIS OR VULVAR VESTIBULITIS

This is an important, frequently misdiagnosed or missed condition that causes pain on sexual intercourse, particularly penetration. Tampons may also be too uncomfortable to use. The condition presents as small areas of localised erythema (Plate 6.5) and tenderness at the introitus, classically over the vestibular gland openings at the 5 o'clock and 7 o'clock positions. Some form of magnification, such as a colposcope, may be required to see the lesions adequately. The cause of focal vulvitis is currently unknown. A variety of treatments have been used in this condition with, unfortunately, often poor response. These include topical steroids, intralesional triamcinolone, cryotherapy and laser ablation. Modified vestibulectomy has produced good results in some studies but patients need to be selected with care.

Vulval burning

'Essential vulvodynia' is the term used to describe symptoms of vulval burning with a normal appearing epithelium. Pudendal neuralgia is an important cause with some patients demonstrating diminished sensation in the sacral sensory distribution. A recent paper reported an association between benign sacral meningeal cysts and genital pain and burning in both men and women. Diagnosis was made by magnetic resonance imaging of the lumbosacral spine.

In the majority of patients, however, no obvious physical cause can be found in which case psychological issues should be considered and addressed.

Management may include the use of 'pain modifiers', such as low to medium dose amitriptyline, prothiaden or fluoxetine, hypnosis, acupuncture, TENS or caudal injection.

Other vulval conditions

VULVAL OEDEMA

The lax vulval skin is prone to oedema and is particularly associated with infections such as herpes, candidiasis and syphilis, although the latter is rare in the U.K. nowadays. Oedema is an occasional feature of contact dermatitis and has been reported following intercourse in women with semen allergy. Vulval oedema may be a presenting sign of Crohn's disease and intrapelvic pathology.

ANGIOKERATOMATA

These small lesions usually appear on the labia majora as tiny, often multiple, bright red vascular spots (Plate 6.6). They may increase in number and size with age and are harmless.

MELANOCYTIC NAEVI

These may appear anywhere on the vulva or perineum and have the same characteristics as naevi elsewhere on the body.

Important management points for vulval disease

- Vulval moistness may increase the risk of secondary infection with yeasts or bacteria. Advise patients to dry the skin thoroughly after washing, if possible with a hair dryer on cool setting. Avoid tight clothing and try to ventilate the area as much as sociably possible.
- Even with careful attention, secondary infection of genital dermatoses may occur. Treatment with a combined anti-infective and steroidal preparation should be considered.
- Although creams are often easier to apply to the genital epithelium they may sting a little more than ointments.
- Soap, bubble-bath, shower gel and feminine washes should be avoided. Many women find aqueous cream or emulsifying ointment useful as soap substitutes for cleansing. Applying cold cream from the refrigerator can be particularly soothing.
- Vulval biopsy may be required to accurately diagnose skin dermatoses. The application of lignocaine + prilocaine cream prior to injecting local anaesthetic makes this a painless and generally well-tolerated procedure.

– All painful vulval conditions have the potential to cause a secondary vaginismus that can often persist after the original complaint has settled. This will require appropriate treatment and follow-up.

– Vulval disease is often chronic and inevitably affects relationships and leads to a degree of psychological morbidity. Psychological support is therefore an important part of the management of these patients and should be considered along with treatment aimed at the physical component of the condition.

– The diagnosis and management of vulval disease can be difficult and may, in some cases, require the assistance of a clinician with a specific interest in the vulva. Many hospitals now run 'vulva clinics' where specialists in GU medicine, dermatology and gynaecology offer a combined opinion. This is the ideal approach to vulval disease.

CHAPTER 9

Frequency–dysuria syndrome

Frequency and dysuria in the female are usually due to:

- cystitis
- urethritis/urethral syndrome
- vulvitis.

Women with vulvitis will often complain of more generalised vulval irritation or soreness in addition to dysuria. It is impossible to distinguish between cystitis and urethritis/urethral syndrome by symptoms alone. As a useful rule of thumb, if the MSU is negative or shows sterile pyuria, consider urethritis/urethral syndrome.

Cystitis

In cystitis, the MSU should contain $> 10^5$ uropathogens per ml. This criterion was originally established for diagnosing acute pyelonephritis and several studies have since suggested that a lower bacterial count of between 10^3 and 10^5 per ml indicates bladder infection. Recent studies have reported that between one-third to one-half of women with bacterial cystitis have 'low-count' bacteruria. The commonest causes of cystitis are *Escherichia coli*, *Staphylococcus saprophyticus*, *Proteus mirabilis*, *Klebsiella pneumoniae* and *Enterobacter* spp.

Urethritis/urethral syndrome

Women with frequency and dysuria and urine containing $< 10^3$ uropathogens per ml with or without pyuria are usually diagnosed as having 'urethral syndrome'. Some will have a true urethritis that may be diagnosed by finding polymorphs on a Gram-stained urethral smear, an investigation routinely performed in GU medicine.

Chlamydia trachomatis is the most important organism to consider. Appropriate swabs should be taken from the cervix in addition to the urethra as infection at both sites is common.

Although some studies have suggested that fastidious bacteria colonising the vulval vestibule, such as lactobacilli and diphtheroids, may occasionally infect the urethra and produce frequency and dysuria, this continues to be a topic of debate.

Other causes of urethral syndrome include:

— gonorrhoea (very unusual to present with frequency–dysuria as the only symptoms)
— herpes (usually associated with vulval or periurethral ulceration)
— trichomoniasis (usually associated with an increased vaginal discharge)
— human papillomavirus infection (a small intrameatal/distal urethral genital wart).

INVESTIGATION OF FREQUENCY–DYSURIA

Dipstix testing and looking at the urine are useful first-line tests. Cystitis is highly unlikely if the urine looks clear and dipstix testing is negative for nitrites, leucocytes, blood and protein.

As a general rule, consider sending an MSU for microscopy and culture if dipstix testing is positive for nitrites, leucocytes, blood or protein although bear in mind that contamination with vaginal discharge may yield positive dipstix results for leucocytes, protein or blood. Women with recurrent symptoms should ideally have tests repeated at the onset of each symptomatic episode.

If these tests prove negative consider:

— checking for chlamydial infection by taking urethral AND cervical swabs (if either are positive, sexual partners MUST be assessed)
— taking a vaginal swab for *Trichomonas vaginalis* and *Candida* culture
— referring to GU medicine for colposcopic examination of the urethral meatus, distal urethra and periurethral area for evidence of tiny genital warts, small herpetic ulcers or a localised area of vulvitis. Examination should be performed when symptoms are present.

RECURRENT FREQUENCY–DYSURIA

— Women with recurrent episodes of proven cystitis should be referred

to urology for investigation of urinary tract pathology.
— Some women with a 'low-set', almost intravaginal urethral meatus are prone to recurrent postcoital cystitis. Attacks may be prevented by urinating directly after intercourse or by using prophylactic single dose antibiotics pre- or postcoitus.
— Advise wiping from 'front-to-back' after defecation.
— Consider a 10–14 day course of a tetracycline. The currently available tests for chlamydial infection are not 100% sensitive.
— Urethral dilatation or urethrotomy will benefit some women.

A number of women suffer chronic urinary symptoms for which no obvious cause can be found. Underlying psychological issues should be carefully sought and discussed openly with the patient. Suggesting that symptoms are 'in the mind' is usually unhelpful whereas an approach that recognises the symptoms as real and attempts to help the patient to 'de-focus' the mind from the urinary tract by way of hypnosis, meditation or low-moderate dose antidepressants, as used for chronic pain relief, may prove helpful.

CHAPTER 10

Pelvic pain

Women with acute, severe pelvic pain are most appropriately assessed by a gynaecologist.

Chronic or recurrent pelvic pain can be notoriously difficult to diagnose and manage and although many women will eventually require a gynaecological assessment, GU medicine can play an important role in assessing patients for evidence of genital infection. Referral to GU medicine may therefore be an appropriate first step for women with pelvic discomfort or pain and if no evidence of infection is found gynaecological referral should then be considered.

Pelvic inflammatory disease (PID) is difficult to diagnose without the aid of laparoscopy and many women are unfortunately labelled as having PID on insufficient clinical grounds. This can lead to a great deal of anxiety, particularly regarding infertility. It is impractical to offer laparoscopy to all women with pelvic pain and if PID is considered a possible diagnosis then the uncertainty of the diagnosis should be discussed with the patient, the appropriate genital swabs taken, appropriate antibiotics prescribed, male sexual partners assessed for asymptomatic urethritis and the patient reassessed after treatment.

Chlamydia trachomatis is the commonest cause of PID in the U.K. and although many women will present with increased vaginal discharge and pelvic discomfort/pain, there is now good evidence to suggest that *Chlamydia* can produce subclinical pelvic infection. As with classical PID, subclinical infection may cause tubal damage and subsequent infertility.

Gonorrhoea has become less common in the U.K. in recent years but the diagnosis must be considered in all women with presumed pelvic infection.

DIAGNOSIS AND MANAGEMENT OF PELVIC INFLAMMATORY DISEASE

1. The following swabs should be taken:
   (a) Vaginal and cervical swabs for Gram staining and microscopy. Unfortunately these are rarely performed in settings other than GU medicine clinics in the U.K. Most PID results from an ascending lower genital tract infection, so there is often evidence of an abnormal vaginal microflora, such as bacterial vaginosis, or of a cervicitis. Mucopurulent cervical secretions provide clinical evidence of cervicitis; however, this is not always easy to assess unless there is excellent lighting and an experienced eye (see also p. 20). Confirmation can be made by examining a Gram-stained smear of cervical secretions by microscopy: the presence of >40 polymorphs per HPF is highly suggestive of cervicitis. A normal lactobacilli-predominant vaginal flora and the absence of cervicitis makes PID a less likely diagnosis.
   (b) Cervical swabs (NOT vaginal) for *Chlamydia* detection and *Neisseria gonorrhoeae* culture. Remember that organisms may be present in the uterus and fallopian tubes in spite of negative cervical cultures.
2. A raised ESR and peripheral white blood cell count are often present in acute PID but are non-specific and therefore provide little clinical guidance.
3. Remember that the most important differential diagnoses for acute PID are acute appendicitis and ectopic pregnancy. Other conditions which may mimic PID include endometriosis, corpus luteum bleeding, urinary tract infection, mesenteric lymphadenitis and ovarian tumour. The more common differential diagnoses of chronic pelvic pain include endometriosis, irritable bowel syndrome and pelvic congestion.
4. Treatment of PID should include antibiotics active against *Chlamydia*, anaerobes and the gonococcus.
   Possible oral combinations include:
   – Doxycycline 100 mg bd + co-amoxiclav 500 mg tds
     or
   – Doxycycline 100 mg bd + metronidazole 400 mg bd + ciprofloxacin 500 mg bd
     or
   – Doxycycline 100 mg bd + metronidazole 400 mg bd + cephalexin 500 mg qds.
   At least 2–3 weeks of antichlamydial and antianaerobic treatment are recommended. Ciprofloxacin or cephalexin may be stopped after 1

week. There is currently no evidence to suggest that treatment with non-steroidal anti-inflammatory drugs reduces the risk of tubal scarring.

5. Advise bed rest and analgesia as required.

6. It is imperative that sexual partners are assessed for evidence of urethritis and treated, otherwise recurrence is likely. Further attacks of PID increase the chances of infertility: following three episodes of PID there is a more than 50% chance of infertility. Urethritis is frequently asymptomatic in male contacts of women with PID, a point worth stressing to the patient.

7. A number of women suffer chronic pelvic pain for which no obvious cause can be found. Underlying psychological issues should be carefully sought and discussed openly with the patient. Suggesting that symptoms are 'in the mind' is usually unhelpful whereas an approach that recognises the symptoms as real and attempts to help the patient 'de-focus' by way of hypnosis, meditation or low-dose antidepressants, as used for chronic pain relief, may prove helpful.

CHAPTER 11

Cytology and colposcopy

Cervical cancer is in most cases a preventable disease and cervical cytology is an effective method of screening for abnormalities that have the potential to progress to cancer. There is a degree of regional variation, but smears are frequently recommended every 3 years for women under 35 years of age and every 5 years after that age. If a woman is having her first smear at 35 years or above, her second smear should be performed after 3 years. Repeat smears are not generally recommended for women over the age of 65 years unless there is a history of not previously having smears performed.

Most of us will have passed through undergraduate training without proper instruction on how to take a cervical smear and occasionally the basic principles are forgotten, even by the most experienced clinician. There are three important points to consider.

1. To obtain a 'good' smear the cervix must be well visualised. This is an obvious point but not always followed. The following guidelines may help to make the procedure a little easier for both patient and practitioner.
   (a) Try to relax the patient.
   (b) Warm the speculum.
   (c) Use an appropriately sized speculum. A nulliparous woman in her early twenties usually requires a smaller speculum than a 40-year-old woman with five children. A very long speculum is occasionally required; it is well worthwhile keeping one or two in the surgery.
   (d) Insert the speculum gently and open slowly. A heavy hand leads to discomfort and may deter the patient from attending for gynaecological examinations in the future.
   (e) Good lighting is essential.
2. Cervical dysplasia and neoplasia usually originate in the 'transformation zone' or 'squamo-columnar junction' (see Fig. 11.1). To help adequately sample this area a range of shapes of cervical spatulae and brushes are

(a) Ectopy or ectropion present

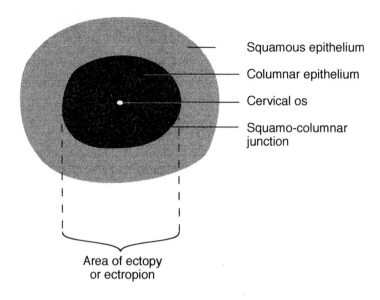

Squamous epithelium

Columnar epithelium

Cervical os

Squamo-columnar junction

Area of ectopy or ectropion

(b) No ectopy or ectropion

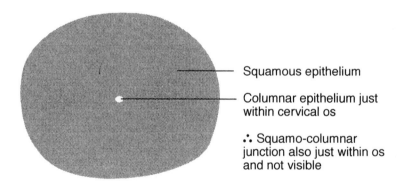

Squamous epithelium

Columnar epithelium just within cervical os

∴ Squamo-columnar junction also just within os and not visible

Fig. 11.1 Cervical squamo-columnar junction or 'transformation' zone.

available (Fig. 11.2). Pick the most appropriate device for the individual cervix. As a basic guide, if there is no obvious ectropion or ectopy the squamo-columnar junction will be just at or inside the cervical os, then an Aylesbury spatula or 'Cervex' sampler should provide an adequate sample. A cervical brush can also be used but ideally this should be in conjunction with a sample obtained by spatula. A 'brush only' sample often contains too few squamous cells for adequate assessment. Brush

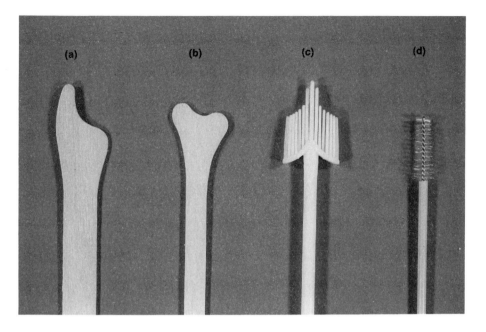

Fig. 11.2 Cervical spatulae and brushes. (a) Aylesbury spatula; (b) Ayre's spatula; (c) Cervex® brush; (d) cervical brush.

and spatula samples may be spread on to different halves of the same slide. Take the brush sample last as the cells tend to dry out quickly, roll the brush over the slide and fix immediately. Combined 'brush and spatula' samples are usually required after cervical surgery (e.g. LLETZ (large loop excision of the transformation zone), laser, cone biopsy).

An Aylesbury spatula should also be suitable if there is a small ectropion whereas an Ayre's spatula is probably best reserved for the cervix with a moderately sized or large ectropion. The entire squamo-columnar junction must be sampled which in some women requires quite firm pressure if the posterior aspect of the junction is to be reached. Two or three 360 degree turns usually picks up sufficient material combined with a lateral sweep if the ectropion is particularly large. Spread the material evenly over the microscope slide and fix immediately. If there is only a scanty amount of material on the slide, resample with a 'Cervex' brush or one of the newer plastic/foam bendable devices, again remembering to aim for the squamo-columnar junction.

Mention on the cytology form if you have used a cervical brush because it often picks up glandular components that can give the cytologist the false impression of cervical pathology.

Cervical smears are best performed at mid-cycle but the opportunity should not be missed to take a smear at other times, except during menstruation.

3. A large number of women think that the main objective of cervical cytology is to detect cervical cancer and there are probably an appreciable number who are deterred from having cervical smears because of this. The misconception is reinforced by using the term 'cancer smear' and by telling women with negative smears that there was 'no evidence of cancer/malignancy'. When a subsequent smear shows 'slight abnormalities' very reasonably the thought of cancer will come to mind and generate a great deal of unnecessary anxiety. Our health education message needs to change to ensure that women fully understand the purpose of cervical smears, i.e. to detect changes in the cells of the cervix which may, in a small number of cases, progress over many years to cancer. Greater emphasis should be made of the likelihood of minor abnormalities returning to normal and of the fact that if these minor changes persist or progress then treatment can be initiated and so prevent the development of cancer at a later date. Unfortunately, because there is currently no way of determining which changes will return to normal and which will progress, a number of women undergo unnecessary treatment. Continued surveillance of minor cervical pathology by cytology and colposcopy does cause anxiety and many women therefore prefer to opt for treatment.

Smear report: terminology briefly explained

Cervical smear terminology is rather complicated and can be very difficult to explain in simple lay terms. It is well worthwhile spending a little time discussing the possible results and their significance with the patient at the time of taking the smear and providing an information leaflet to take away. This may help to reduce anxiety should the smear need repeating at an earlier time interval or should there be a need to refer on for colposcopy.

INADEQUATE SPECIMEN

There are a number of reasons why a smear is considered inadequate for assessment and some of these may be rectified before the smear is taken or sent to the laboratory.

(1) 'Scanty specimen'. As mentioned above, if there is little material on

the slide repeat the sampling with a Cytobrush or Cervex brush. This should be mentioned on the smear form.

(2) 'Blood stained specimen: too many red blood cells for adequate assessment'. Some cervices bleed profusely as the smear is taken. This may indicate cervicitis or too firm a pressure when sampling. If there is some cervical mucus on the slide it is probably worthwhile sending the specimen to the laboratory. If the smear appears to be purely blood repeat at a later date. If bleeding occurs again check for cervical infection, in particular *Chlamydia*. Consider treating with a tetracycline or alternatively refer to GU medicine for assessment.

(3) 'Excessive bacteria'. This is usually due to bacterial vaginosis, a condition caused by an overgrowth of various bacteria, in particular *Gardnerella vaginalis*, *Mycoplasma hominis*, *Bacteroides* spp. and other anaerobes (see p. 9). If these cover the specimen the cervical cells are obscured and therefore cannot be properly assessed. Bacterial vaginosis usually only requires treatment if there are symptoms of vaginal discharge; however, when the condition interferes with cervical cytology consider treating before resampling.

(4) 'Excess pus cells/polymorphs'. This may result from cervicitis or vaginitis. If you think clinically there is a vaginitis, take a swab for *Trichomonas* and *Candida* culture and treat with an antifungal. If there is clinical evidence of cervicitis, and this may be very difficult to assess, check for cervical pathogens such as *Chlamydia* and *Neisseria gonorrhoeae*. Ideally patients with presumed cervicitis should be referred to GU medicine for assessment.

Candida may be seen on a cervical smear but it only usually interferes with assessment if there are excessive numbers of pus cells or candidal pseudohyphae and spores. Treatment is only necessary if symptoms are present or if the smear cannot be adequately assessed.

Trichomonas vaginalis may also be seen on a cervical smear; however, it is always worth confirming with vaginal culture as false positive results may occur with cytology.

(5) 'No endocervical component present'. There is continuing debate as to whether an adequate smear needs to contain endocervical and/or metaplastic cells. In fact, the only smears that can be judged with certainty as adequate are those containing abnormal cells. The presence of endocervical/metaplastic cells suggests that the squamo-columnar junction has been sampled, either partly or fully. If no endocervical component is present in a woman's first smear, consider repeating in 3 months. If previous smears have been negative, consider repeating in 1 year.

(6) 'Poor spreading of material' or 'poor fixation'. Always remember to spread the sample as evenly as possible over the slide and fix immediately before it air dries.

INFLAMMATORY SMEAR

Some cytology laboratories use this term to mean excessive pus cells suggesting inflammation and possible infection. More commonly, however, it refers to nuclear abnormalities insufficient to be termed dyskaryosis. If there is clinical evidence of cervicitis or the patient has noticed an increased discharge, check for infection (*Chlamydia* and gonorrhoea), either in the surgery or preferably refer to GU medicine. If the cervix looks normal, repeat the smear in 3–6 months time. The inflammatory changes often resolve without antibiotic treatment. If inflammatory changes persist, check for infection as mentioned above and consider prescribing a course of tetracycline or erythromycin. If no infective cause is found and there is no improvement with antibiotics refer for colposcopy.

HUMAN PAPILLOMAVIRUS INFECTION (see also Chapter 18)

Human papillomavirus (HPV) is the commonest sexually transmitted viral infection in the developed world. Although HPV causes genital warts most HPV infection is 'subclinical'. Studies using extremely sensitive methods for detecting viral DNA (polymerase chain reaction) have identified low levels of HPV in many sexually active women. This may either clear with time or persist indefinitely. Subclinical HPV infection can sometimes be diagnosed on cervical cytology by identifying cells called 'koilocytes'. The cells have a prominent nucleus and the cytoplasm contains a large perinuclear halo. These appearances are considered pathognomonic of HPV infection. Certain HPV types, in particular types 16 and 18, are strongly associated with high grade cervical dysplasia (CIN (cervical intraepithelial neoplasia) II/III) and neoplasia. For this reason, women with evidence of HPV on cervical cytology require careful follow-up and the usual recommendation is to repeat the smear after 6 months.

BORDERLINE NUCLEAR CHANGES

This suggests nuclear abnormalities that are insufficient to be termed dyskaryosis. Borderline nuclear changes may be found in the presence of HPV infection, in association with inflammatory changes or in women with an IUCD. A borderline smear should be repeated in 6 months; if borderline changes persist, refer for colposcopy.

DYSKARYOSIS

This means that the cell nucleus is abnormal. There are three grades of dyskaryosis: mild, moderate and severe. The equivalent histological terms are mild, moderate and severe dysplasia or CIN I, II and III. The concept of dyskaryosis is very difficult to explain in lay terms. The term 'pre-cancer', although theoretically correct, is a little too dramatic and often causes anxiety. An 'abnormality of the cells which is not cancerous but which may in a small number of women progress to cancer over many years' is rather wordy but fairly accurate and with emphasis on 'not', 'may', 'small' and 'many' tends to avoid leaving the patient with a feeling of pending doom. It can of course be difficult to achieve the right balance between causing undue anxiety and producing excessive complacency. Tailoring the wording to the individual patient is essential.

Women with smears showing moderate or severe dyskaryosis should be referred immediately for colposcopy. There is still debate as to whether women with mild dyskaryosis require immediate colposcopy or whether the smear should be repeated at 6 months and colposcopy reserved for women with persisting abnormalities. Although the evidence for immediate colposcopy is highly persuasive such a policy would have important practical and financial implications. One must therefore be guided by local guidelines.

Colposcopy

A number of studies have reported high levels of anxiety among women attending colposcopy clinics. Providing accurate information and carefully explaining how colposcopy is performed and what is likely to happen undoubtedly reduces the anxiety. Most women will be referred for colposcopy if mild cytological abnormalities persist (e.g. borderline changes or mild dyskaryosis) or if there is a single smear showing moderate or severe dyskaryosis. The following points should be covered at the time of referral.

1. Explain that the colposcope is purely a magnifying system which enables the cervix to be examined in greater detail. It is worth emphasising that the colposcope does not enter the vagina and the procedure is

rather like having a cervical smear. A weak vinegar solution (usually 5% acetic acid) is used to help show up abnormal areas on the cervix and this does very occasionally sting a little.

2. If an abnormality is seen a biopsy will be taken, usually without local anaesthesia. Some women feel a short sharp pain as the biopsy is taken while others find this only mildly uncomfortable, likening the sensation to a firm pinch. A few colposcopists inject a small amount of local anaesthetic prior to biopsy. This is very slightly uncomfortable but does ensure that the rest of the procedure is virtually painless.

3. After a biopsy has been taken some women experience period-like pains that may persist for several hours. This is usually relieved by paracetamol or ibuprofen.

4. There may be spotting of blood for a couple of days after taking a biopsy. Sexual intercourse should be avoided for a few days until healing occurs.

5. The patient is usually asked to return in a couple of weeks for the result of histology and further management is discussed at that time. Some colposcopists prefer to 'see and treat' on the first clinic attendance which usually involves performing a LLETZ.

6. Most colposcopy clinics provide information leaflets for patients which are sent out with the appointment. Providing information in the GP surgery at the time of referral is probably more appropriate and is best approached by having your local colposcopy clinic send details of their current management policy.

TREATMENT OF CERVICAL INTRAEPITHELIAL NEOPLASIA

Although this will vary from unit to unit, many now use LLETZ in preference to laser ablation or cold coagulation. This is usually performed under local anaesthesia and has been shown to be a safe and effective procedure with no subsequent effect on menstruation or fertility. Repeat colposcopy is usually recommended 1 year after treatment and annual smears for 5 years.

CHAPTER 12

Contraception and genital tract infection

Many GPs provide contraceptive advice to youngsters who have recently become sexually active or who are considering starting sexual relationships. In the U.K., the median age of first sexual intercourse is now 17 years for both sexes and just over a quarter of men and just under a fifth of women have had intercourse before the age of 16 years. The time between first sexual experience and first intercourse is currently 4 years for men and 3 years for women (i.e. age of first sexual experience is 13 years for men and 14 years for women). Approximately half of those having intercourse before the age of 16 years use no contraception and about one-third of sexually active teenagers fail to use contraception at the time of first intercourse. The U.K. has one of the highest teenage conception rates in Western Europe, with just over one-half of pregnancies in under 16-year-olds ending in termination. These data emphasise the importance of providing the young and sexually active with easy access to contraception. The opportunity should also be taken to discuss other sexual health matters, in particular how to avoid acquiring sexually transmitted infections. This chapter looks at the issue of contraception and STDs in a little more detail.

Condoms

Laboratory studies have shown that latex condoms are effective mechanical barriers against hepatitis B virus, HIV, cytomegalovirus, herpes simplex virus and *Chlamydia*.

Epidemiological studies have shown that correct and consistent use of condoms protect against gonorrhoea, NGU and HIV infection. No relationship has been found between condom use and HPV infection. To be protective the condom must cover that part of the genital tract which is infected or likely to become infected, for example the cervix in the female and the urethra in the male. Protection is less likely for infections that may affect the vulva and perineum or the epithelium beyond the penile shaft, for example genital herpes and HPV infection.

There are a few points worth emphasising. Firstly, condoms must be used correctly, i.e. placed on to the penis before genital contact and unrolled fully to cover as much of the penis as possible. Teated condoms should have the air squeezed from the end as they are unrolled. Many youngsters do not know how to use a condom, particularly when they are being used for the first time. Condom manufacturers are usually happy to provide plastic demonstration models. These should be considered essential equipment for all GP surgeries and clinics that provide contraceptive or sexual health advice.

Condoms do occasionally split or slip off the penis during intercourse. Individuals who are particularly prone to these mishaps should check that they are fully unrolling the condom and that fingernails are not damaging the latex. In addition, some non-water based lubricants and various vaginal preparations may damage latex and therefore should NOT be used in conjunction with either the condom or diaphragm. There preparations include: baby oil, petroleum jelly, vaseline, 2% clindamycin cream, Eco-statin, Fungilin, Gyno-Daktarin, Gyno-Pevaryl, Monistat, Nizoral, Nys-tatin cream, Ortho Dienoestrol, Ortho Gynest, Premarin, Sultrin, Witep-sol-based suppositories, hair conditioner, skin softener, bath oil, massage oil, body oil, suntan oil, lipstick, cooking oil, margarine, butter, salad cream, cream and ice cream!

A tremendous effort has been put into condom marketing in recent years and the larger manufacturers now provide a wide range of shapes, colours and flavours. Apparently mint and Pina Colada flavoured condoms are particularly well accepted. Occasionally low standard condoms find their way on to the market and for this reason only brands which display the British Standards 'Kite Mark' should be used.

A common reason given by men for not using condoms is decreased sensitivity and hence reduced sexual pleasure. A technique termed 'gel charging' does appear to heighten the sexual experience for some men and therefore may help to encourage condom use. This involves placing a small amount (e.g. a teaspoonful) of lubricant or spermicidal gel into the end of a condom before placing onto the penis. Contoured and flared condoms apparently give the most effective results.

Diaphragm

Less information is available regarding the diaphragm, but the small number of studies which have been performed do show that this form of contraception provides women with protection against gonorrhoea and other cervical infections.

Diaphragm use does appear to increase the risk of urinary tract infection.

Spermicides

Nonoxynol-9 is a commonly used spermicide that also inhibits the growth of several sexually transmitted organisms. These include *Neisseria gonor-rhoeae*, *Chlamydia trachomatis*, *Treponema pallidum*, herpes simplex virus, cytomegalovirus and HIV. It appears to have no action against HPV. Although many condoms are impregnated with spermicide it is uncertain whether the amount present would be sufficient to kill these pathogens if the condom split. There is also some concern that frequent use of nonoxynol-9 may produce vulvovaginal inflammation and possibly ulceration. These adverse reactions are of relevance to women having intercourse several times a day and are probably not applicable to the general sexually active population. Epidemiological studies on the use of spermicides have documented a protective effect against gonorrhoea, trichomoniasis and possibly *Chlamydia* and HIV. There appears to be no effect on bacterial vaginosis or candidiasis.

The 'female condom'

The female condom, known in the U.K. as Femidom, is made from polyurethane. It has been shown in the laboratory to act as a complete barrier to cytomegalovirus, HIV and to bacteriophages smaller than HIV and hepatitis B. The vaginal flora remains unchanged after repeated use and there is no evidence of an irritant effect on the vagina. A pregnancy rate of 2.6% during 6 months' use has been reported for 'perfect users'. Femidom is not acceptable to all women. It can be difficult to insert and occasionally the device can be pushed into the vagina or slip out. Hopefully, design modification will eventually resolve these problems. Unlike most male condoms, the lubricant on female condoms does not contain a spermicide.

Intrauterine contraceptive device

The risk of PID among IUCD users has been generally overstated. There is a transient risk of developing infection at the time of or just after insertion that may be partly related to the degree of experience of the clinician fitting the device. PID affecting a women with an IUCD is often more severe clinically.

Hormonal contraceptives

Hormonal contraceptives have been shown to protect against PID and may reduce the degree of tubal inflammation if infection develops. Although some earlier studies did show an association between oral contraceptive use and chlamydial cervicitis this has not been confirmed by more recent work. *Chlamydia* appears to be more frequently isolated from women with ectropion, irrespective of the method of contraception used.

Important points

1. An ideal approach to contraception for the woman who is not in a steady relationship or who may frequently change sexual partners or who cannot guarantee the fidelity of her partner is to consider using both condoms and hormonal contraception. The favoured method of hormonal contraception is usually the oral contraceptive pill. This approach provides optimal protection against STDs and pregnancy.
2. All women starting oral or barrier contraception should receive information on emergency postcoital contraception. In particular, they need to know where emergency contraception is available and understand that it is appropriate to use 'pills' up to 3 days and an IUCD up to 5 days after unprotected intercourse. The term 'morning after pill' gives the wrong message and should no longer be used. If unprotected intercourse was with a 'new' partner the possibility of acquiring a sexually transmitted infection should be discussed and referral to GU medicine advised. Women with a clinical suspicion or at risk for genital infection should ideally be screened for, in particular, *Chlamydia*, gonorrhoea and bacterial vaginosis and receive a course of tetracycline and metronidazole or co-amoxiclav prior to emergency IUCD insertion. Liaison with colleagues in GU medicine is to be recommended.

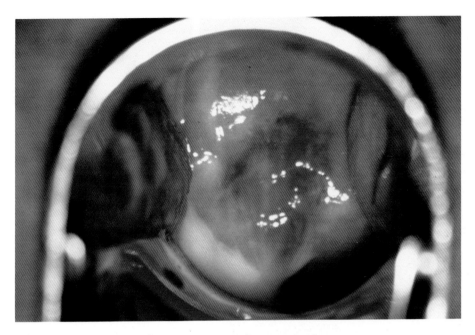

6.1 Cervicitis. Mucopurulent secretions pooling in speculum.

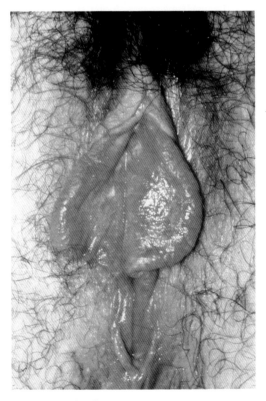

6.2 Candidal vulvitis.

Facing p.50

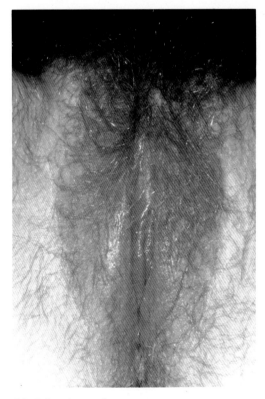

6.3 Seborrhoeic dermatitis.

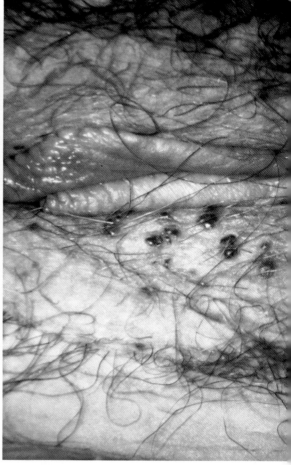

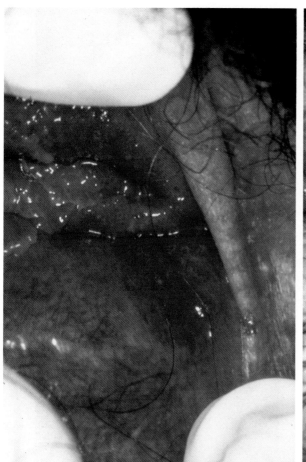

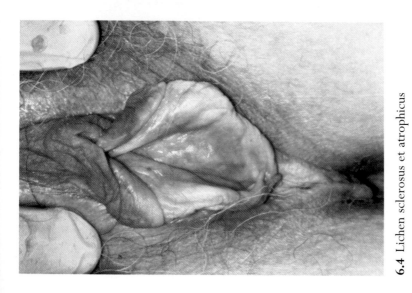

6.4 Lichen sclerosus et atrophicus

6.5 (top right) Focal vulvitis or vulvar vestibulitis. Small area of erythema seen at the introitus at 7 o'clock position.

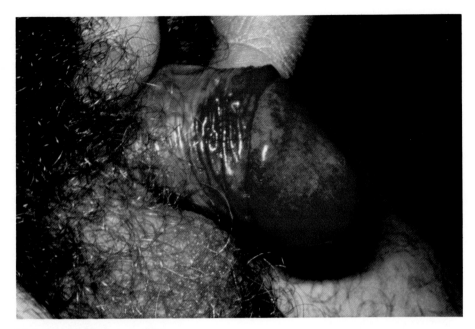

16.1 Candidal balanoposthitis.

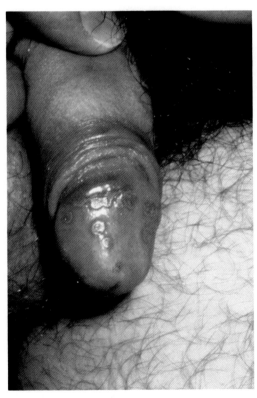

16.2 Circinate balanitis.

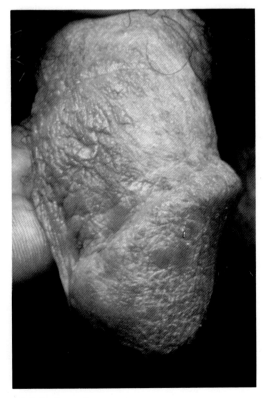

16.3 Lichen planus.

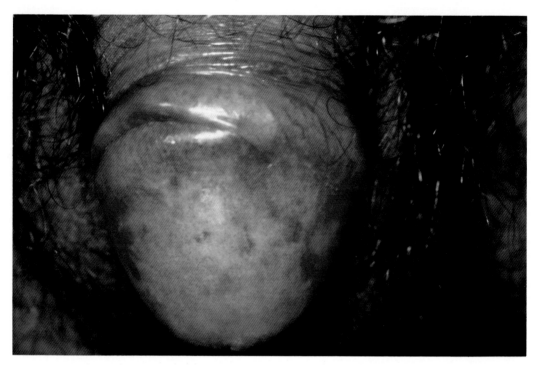

16.4 Lichen sclerosus et atrophicus.

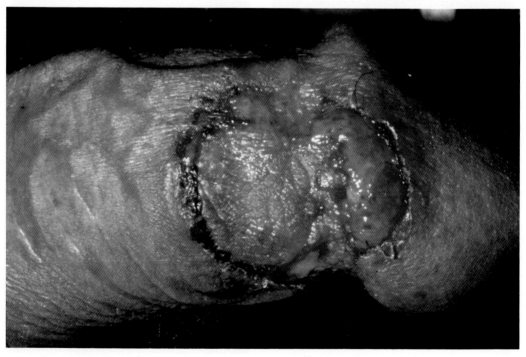

16.5 Fixed drug eruption.

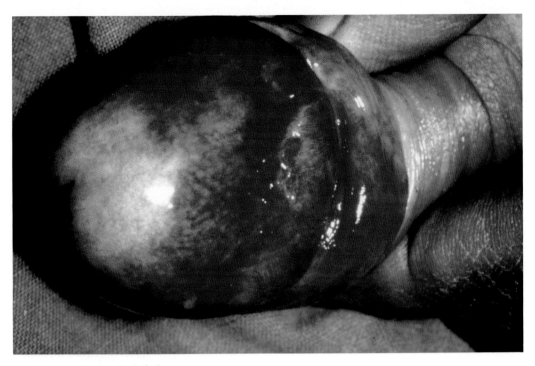

16.6 Zoon's balanitis.

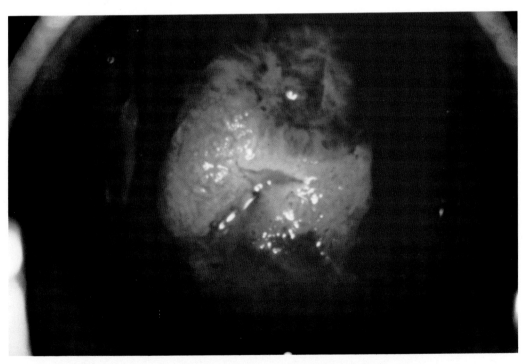

18.1 Cervical warts with surrounding areas of 'acetowhitening' (i.e. whitening of the epithelium following the application of 5% acetic acid solution). Biopsy of this area revealed CIN III (see Chapter 11).

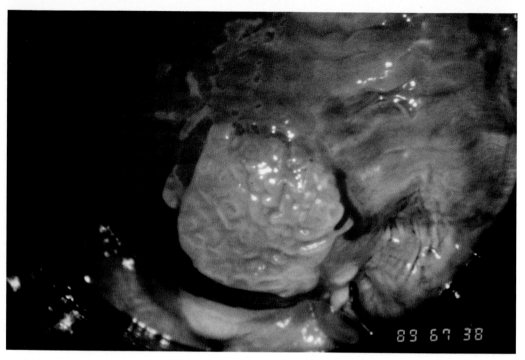

18.2 Anal warts with adjacent areas of 'acetowhitening'. Biopsy of this area revealed severe anal dysplasia or anal intraepithelial neoplasia (AIN) III.

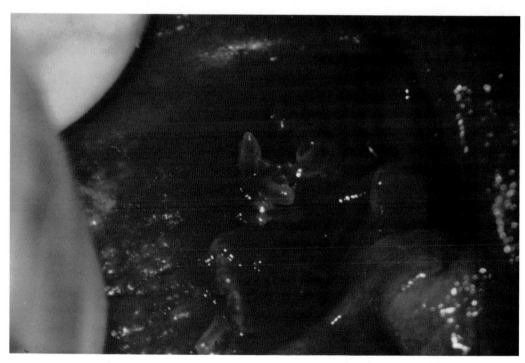

18.3 Vulval micropapillae.

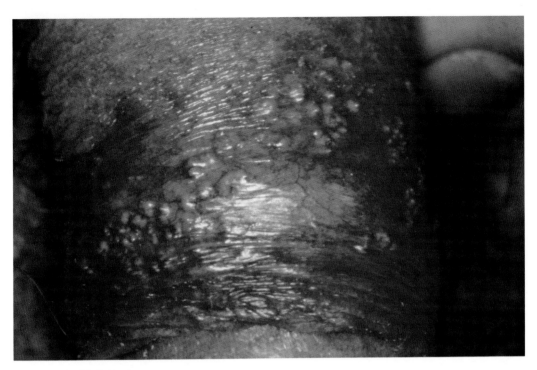

18.4 Fordyce spots.

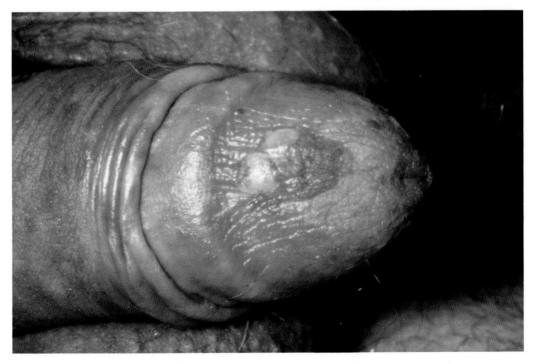

18.5 Condylomata lata. A feature of secondary syphilis.

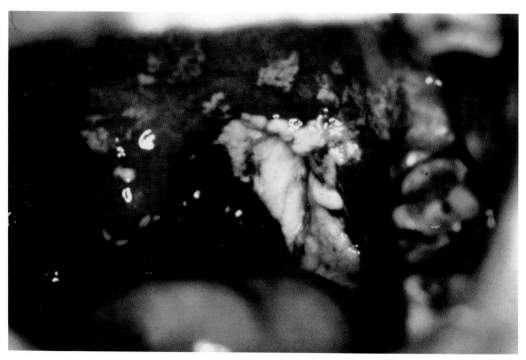

20.1 Oral candidiasis.

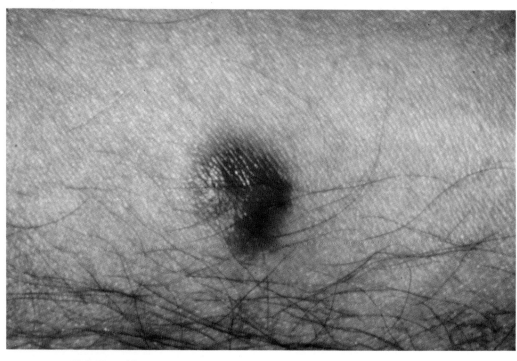

20.2 Kaposi's sarcoma.

CHAPTER 13

Dysuria in young men

The commonest cause of dysuria in the young, single, sexually active male is urethritis rather than cystitis.

Urethritis is usually the result of a sexually acquired infection and may be conveniently divided into gonorrhoea or 'gonococcal urethritis' and 'not-gonorrhoea' or 'non-gonococcal urethritis' (NGU). NGU is also known as 'non-specific urethritis' (NSU).

Other symptoms associated with urethritis include urethral discharge, which may not be noticed by the patient, and frequency.

The causes of NGU are:

- *Chlamydia trachomatis* (40–60%); although these cases should be called 'chlamydial urethritis', the term '*Chlamydia*-positive NGU' is often used.
- *Ureaplasma urealyticum* (? 10–20%); there is still some debate concerning the role of ureaplasmas in urethritis.

The following make up only a small percentage of cases, hence most NGU is truly non-specific, i.e. no specific organism can be isolated.

- *Trichomonas vaginalis*
- Herpes simplex virus
- *E. coli* (usually causes cystitis although it has been documented as a cause of urethritis in homosexual men)
- *Mycoplasma genitalium*
- ? Certain anaerobes (e.g. *Bacteroides urealyticus*)
- Traumatic (e.g. postcatheterisation, after pencil or biro insertion)
- Reactive (e.g. postdysenteric Reiter's syndrome may be associated with a urethritis). This is not sexually acquired.

Investigations

To diagnose urethritis the following investigations should be performed:

(1) Urethral swab Gram stain: A small foam swab or plastic loop is inserted into the opened meatus and the distal urethra gently swabbed. Secretions are then transferred on to a microscope slide for Gram staining and microscopy.

   The presence of >4 polymorphs per HPF ($\times 1000$) is diagnostic of urethritis.

(2) Two-glass urine test: The patient is asked to pass the first 20–50 ml of his urinary stream into a glass and the second part of the stream into a second glass (any remaining in the bladder can be directed in to the urinal). The presence of 'threads' or 'specks' of pus in the first glass with a clear second glass indicates an anterior urethritis. Pus in both glasses suggests a posterior urethritis or cystitis. If this is the case, send the first glass or an MSU to the laboratory for culture. Patients with a profuse discharge due to NGU or gonorrhoea may show pus in both glasses; however, this will be much heavier in the first glass.

   Phosphaturia is a common cause of cloudy urine and may be mistaken for pyuria. The addition of acetic acid will rapidly clear the urine if phosphates are present; if the urine remains cloudy then pyuria is the likely cause.

   A rather more scientific method of diagnosing urethritis from the first catch urine is to examine the resuspended urinary sediment under the microscope. The presence of >15 polymorphs in any of five random fields ($\times 400$) indicates a urethritis. Some studies have suggested that examination of the urine may be a more sensitive method of detecting mild urethritis than the urethral Gram stain.

   Cases of mild urethritis may be missed if the patient has recently passed urine before the above investigations are performed. For this reason patients should be asked to hold on to their urine for at least 3 h prior to assessment. If the history is suggestive of urethritis and the initial investigations prove negative, repeat testing should be performed early in the morning, the patient having held on to his urine overnight.

(3) Whenever possible, a urethral swab should also be taken for detection of *Chlamydia*, as occasionally chlamydial infection may be present in the absence of an obvious urethritis. Finding *Chlamydia*, however, does not alter patient management. Tetracycline is first-line treatment for both *Chlamydia*-positive and *Chlamydia*-negative NGU.

(4) Gonococcal urethritis is far less common than NGU, but a urethral swab should be taken for *Neisseria gonorrhoeae* culture. Remember that the gonococcus is particularly delicate and may well not survive an overnight delay before plating on to specific culture media. If gonor-

rhoea is considered a possible diagnosis, the patient should be referred to GU medicine so that swabs may be plated on to the appropriate culture media and incubated prior to transport to the laboratory. The important issue of contact tracing can also be addressed.

(5) Send an MSU or first-catch urine for microscopy and culture if the two-glass urine test suggests posterior urethritis/cystitis or if urine dipstix testing shows the presence of nitrites or blood.

Management of non-gonococcal urethritis

Most GP surgeries do not have access to immediate microscopy and there may be a delay in transporting microbiology specimens to the laboratory; therefore patients with suspected urethritis should be referred to GU medicine for assessment. Urethritis is considered an urgent problem requiring immediate attention. A telephone call to the clinic before sending along the patient is appreciated, however, as most clinics run an appointment system.

First-line treatment for NGU should be a tetracycline for 10–14 days. Oxytetracycline 500 mg qds for 14 days is relatively cheap but compliance may be poor compared with, for example, doxycycline 100 mg bd for 14 days. Erythromycin stearate 500 mg bd for 14 days is a good second-line treatment option.

Single dose azithromycin (1 g), which is active against *Chlamydia*, has been shown to be a useful alternative treatment for NGU.

Sexual partners MUST be assessed and an antibiotic prescribed, namely a tetracycline or erythromycin, even in the absence of infection. The possibility of missing a chlamydial infection with the subsequent development of asymptomatic pelvic infection leading to infertility or ectopic pregnancy warrants such a policy.

Patients should be reassessed following treatment to ensure cure. Resolution of symptoms does not always indicate eradication of infection, hence the importance of repeating tests after treatment. The initial lack of response to treatment may result from poor compliance, reinfection or persistent infection. If persistence is considered likely re-treat with erythromycin (or tetracycline if erythromycin was used as first-line treatment). Reinforce the need to avoid sexual intercourse until partners have been assessed and treated and advise against frequent self-examination, masturbation, spicy foods and excessive alcohol that may aggravate symptoms. A longer course of tetracycline together with metronidazole should be considered if the urethritis persists. Patients with continued symptoms together with objective evidence of urethritis may warrant urethroscopy, urethral ultrasound or a urethrogram.

RECURRENT URETHRITIS

A small number of men suffer repeated episodes of NGU. Some of these will be caused by reinfection from new or previously untreated partners; however, recurrence of urethritis without sexual contact or within a relationship where the sexual partner has received treatment is well recognised. If both partners are monogamous, further treatment of the female partner is probably not warranted. Most clinicians would re-treat the symptomatic male although previous courses of tetracycline and erythromycin significantly reduce the likelihood of ongoing infection.

Some cases of recurrent urethritis are thought to be due to 'immunological hypersensitivity' to a previous infection that results in a persisting inflammatory response.

Management of gonorrhoea

Patients with gonorrhoea should be referred to a GU medicine clinic for treatment, follow-up and contact tracing. If there is a delay before the patient can be seen, consider treating with oral ampicillin 2 g stat plus probenecid 1 g stat and then refer to the GU medicine clinic for follow-up and contact tracing.

Penicillin-resistant gonorrhoea is seen in the U.K., mostly in patients who have had sexual contact with partners from outside the U.K. Although ciprofloxacin 500 mg stat is currently the recommended treatment for penicillin-resistant cases, 4-quinolone-resistant strains have now been reported in the U.K. Most laboratories will provide details of antibiotic sensitivities for their gonococcal isolates.

Prescribing a 10-day course of tetracycline in addition to antigonococcal treatment to cover possible coinfection with *Chlamydia* is to be recommended. Patients should reattend for 'tests of cure' after treatment.

Management of urinary tract infection

As mentioned above, dysuria in the young, sexually active male is more likely to be due to urethritis than to cystitis or urinary tract infection. If a UTI is considered the most likely diagnosis, consider treating with antibiotics which achieve therapeutic concentrations in the prostate (e.g. trimethoprim, norfloxacin, ciprofloxacin).

Men with acute pyelonephritis or who suffer more than one episode of cystitis warrant urological investigation.

Important points

1. Consider a diagnosis of urethritis rather than cystitis in the 'unmarried', sexually active man with dysuria. Urethritis should also be considered in the married or cohabiting man but proceed with a little more caution!

2. Initial investigations should include a urethral Gram stain and two-glass urine test. If both glasses of the two-glass urine test contain pus send off the first glass or an MSU for microscopy and culture and treat as cystitis.

3. If microscopy is unavailable in the GP surgery the patient should be referred to a GU medicine clinic for urgent assessment. Contact tracing can then also be addressed and the opportunity taken to provide health education and information about the condition.

4. Remember that 'contact tracing' or 'partner notification' involves rather more than providing antibiotics for the sexual partner. Partners should be clinically assessed and the possibility of other sexual partners being involved must be addressed.

5. Consider the diagnosis of urethritis in men and women with dysuria and an MSU showing sterile pyuria.

6. NGU is sexually acquired in the majority of cases. Sexual partners MUST be assessed and treated.

7. Although this chapter has focused on men presenting with dysuria, remember that both gonococcal and, in particular, NGU may be asymptomatic. Such individuals may pass on their infection unknowingly to sexual partners and act as important transmitters of disease within the community.

CHAPTER 14

Prostatitis, prostatodynia and haematospermia

Men with 'prostatitis' often find their way to either Urology or GU medicine.

Acute bacterial prostatitis commonly presents with fever, chills, frequency, dysuria or strangury and rectal pain. Examination reveals a tender, swollen prostate gland.

Chronic prostatitis may be more difficult to diagnose clinically. Symptoms usually include perineal or suprapubic discomfort or pain sometimes radiating to the testes and penis. This may be associated with dysuria, frequency and postejaculatory pain. Rectal examination does not usually reveal prostatic tenderness. Chronic abacterial prostatitis is the most common form of prostatitis seen in 'developed' countries. Prostatodynia is the term reserved for men with symptoms suggestive of prostatitis but in whom no evidence of prostatic pathology can be identified.

Other causes of 'prostatitis-like' symptoms:

- Bladder neck dyssynergia (muscular incoordination) may present with frequency, urgency and postmicturition dribbling. Diagnosis is usually by urinary flow studies.
- Pelvic floor tension myalgia presents with frequency, urgency and perineal discomfort and there is pain on palpating the levator ani.
- Pudendal neuralgia may present with perineal and genital pain. Benign sacral meningeal cysts are a recently described cause of genital pain and are best visualised by magnetic resonance imaging (MRI) scanning of the lumbosacral spine. Consider seeking a neurological or urological opinion before embarking on costly investigations.

Investigations

Diagnosing chronic prostatitis can be difficult in general practice. 'Localisation studies' should ideally be performed which involves microscopy of various urine samples pre- and postprostatic massage together with micro-scopy and culture of expressed prostatic secretions. This is summarised in Table 14.1; as you will appreciate, this may be more easily undertaken by a specialist.

It is important to note that chronic abacterial prostatitis differs from chronic bacterial prostatitis in that urine and prostatic secretion cultures are negative. There is an increased number of polymorphs in the expressed prostatic fluid in both conditions.

Transrectal ultrasound may help to diagnose chronic prostatitis and may identify prostatic abscesses; however, this is currently available in only a small number of specialist centres.

Treatment

An urgent urological opinion should be sought for patients with presumed acute prostatitis. The condition is usually caused by the common urinary pathogens (e.g. *E. coli*, *Proteus* spp., *Strep. faecalis*, *Klebsiella* spp., *Pseudomonas* spp.) and is best treated with trimethoprim or a 4-quinolone such as ciprofloxacin or norfloxacin. Intravenous therapy is usually required initially and treatment should continue with oral antibiotics for up to 6 weeks.

Chronic bacterial prostatitis requires an antibiotic that can pass readily into the prostate. A 6–8 week course of ciprofloxacin (500 mg bd) or norfloxacin (400 mg bd) should be considered. Trimethoprim is less effect-ive in this condition.

Patients with chronic abacterial prostatitis and prostatodynia often prove difficult to manage. Although long-term antibiotics are usually ineffective and should strictly only be used if a causative agent is identified, some clinicians recommend a 2–3 week trial of, for example, ciprofloxacin, norfloxacin or doxycycline (100 mg bd).

Non-steroidal anti-inflammatory drugs (NSAIDs) are worth trying, either orally or, possibly preferably, as suppositories together with some form of chronic pain management, such as low to medium dose antide-pressants (e.g. fluoxetine, dothiepin, amitriptyline).

Pollen extract (cernilton) is reported to have anti-inflammatory and anti-adrenergic properties and has been used successfully in some cases of chronic abacterial prostatitis. Treatment may need to be continued for some months.

Microwave hyperthermia to the prostate has also been used with variable success.

Table 14.1. *Diagnosis of prostatitis*

	First catch urine (10 ml)	Second catch or MSU		Expressed prostatic secretions (collected onto slide or into culture bottle)		Urine after prostatic massage	
	Pus cells	Pus cells	Culture	Pus cells	Culture	Pus cells	Culture
Chronic bacterial protatitis	−	+	+	+	+	+	+
Chronic abacterial prostatitis	−	−	−	+	−	+	−
Prostatodynia	−	−	−	−	−	−	−

MSU, mid-stream urine.

Some patients with prostatodynia have a spastic dysfunction of the bladder neck and prostatic urethra and may benefit from an alpha-blocker (e.g. prazosin, terazosin).

In both chronic abacterial prostatitis and prostatodynia, psychological factors should be tactfully sought and addressed and the use of acupuncture, hypnosis or relaxation and visualisation techniques considered. Most importantly, time should be taken to explain that the condition is not precancerous, will not affect fertility and cannot be passed on or acquired through sexual intercourse.

Haematospermia

Blood in the ejaculate is a worrying condition that often raises concerns about cancer or sexually transmitted infection. It is important to distinguish a blood-stained ejaculate from fresh bleeding per urethra (e.g. secondary to intrameatal or distal urethral warts) and traumatic lesions (e.g. a torn frenulum). A careful genital and prostatic examination are therefore required and the appropriate tests taken to check for urethritis, including chlamydial and gonococcal infection, although in the majority of cases these prove negative. The blood pressure should be measured and urinalysis performed to exclude haematuria.

Men under the age of 40 years with no other urinary or genital symptoms require reassurance. The condition may recur but will eventually cease. Men over 40 years of age are at greater risk of having underlying pathology and should undergo further investigation, including transrectal ultrasound.

CHAPTER 15

Scrotal pain

The scrotum and its contents have a complicated nerve supply.

(1) Sympathetic fibres from Tl–L1 supply the testis, vas and epididymis.
(2) Somatic fibres from L1–L2 supply the outer surface of the testis, the tunica vaginalis and the anterior scrotal skin.
(3) Somatic fibres from S2–S3 supply the rest of the scrotal skin.

Scrotal pain may therefore be caused by intrascrotal pathology or result from referred pain from visceral or somatic structures.
   Causes of referred pain include:

(1) Impacted stone in the lower ureter (splanchnic L1)
(2) Small inguinal hernia compressing the genitofemoral nerve
(3) Degenerative lesions of the lower thoracic and upper lumbar spine
(4) Disease of the genital viscera (e.g. prostate, seminal vesicles)
(5) Benign sacral meningeal cysts (see also vulvodynia p. 30)
(6) Aneurysm of the internal iliac artery.

Intrascrotal pathology

EPIDIDYMITIS

The commonest cause of acute scrotal pain in the adult is acute epididymitis. In sexually active men under the age of about 35 years this is usually caused by *Chlamydia trachomatis*. The patient presents with 'pain in the scrotum', but there is often an associated urethritis, which may be asymptomatic. In men over the age of 35 years the commonest causes of epididymitis are the more standard urinary tract pathogens such as *E. coli*, *Pseudomonas* spp., *Klebsiella* spp. and *Proteus* spp.

Investigations

The sexual history may give a clue as to whether the condition is more likely to be sexually or non-sexually transmitted.

In the younger, sexually active single male the initial investigations should include (see also p. 52):

— urethral swab for Gram stain (to look for evidence of urethritis)
— urethral swabs for detection of *Chlamydia* and possibly gonorrhoea culture
— two-glass urine test
— MSU or send off the first glass of the two-glass urine for culture.

In the 'older' age groups, culture of an MSU may be sufficient.

Management

The 'young' sexually active male with epididymitis should ideally be referred to a GU medicine clinic for urgent investigation. If evidence of urethritis is found or a sexually transmitted cause considered likely then treat with an antibiotic active against *Chlamydia*, such as a tetracycline (e.g. oxytetracycline 500 mg qds; doxycycline 100 mg bd). The patient should be reviewed in 1 week or sooner if symptoms worsen. If there is clinical improvement the treatment should be continued for at least 6 weeks. Sexual contacts MUST be assessed, in particular for evidence of chlamydial infection.

If a urinary tract pathogen is considered a more likely cause, treatment with, for example, trimethoprim or norfloxacin should be started while awaiting the results of MSU and sensitivity tests.

Many patients find a scrotal support helpful in addition to simple analgesia.

If there is any doubt about the diagnosis an urgent urological opinion should be sort to exclude torsion of the testis.

TESTICULAR TORSION

Just under 50% of men with testicular torsion give a history of previous brief episodes of scrotal discomfort. All patients with a suspected torsion should be referred urgently for a urological opinion with the view to emergency exploration of the scrotum.

ORCHITIS

This may affect one or both testes and in this country is most commonly associated with mumps. Testicular atrophy develops in approximately 15% of adults following severe mumps orchitis. More unusual causes of orchitis include infectious mononucleosis, coxsackie B virus infection and dengue fever.

TUMOUR

Approximately 10% of testicular tumours present as a painful swelling and may be initially misdiagnosed as epididymitis. Scrotal ultrasound is an extremely useful investigation for determining the cause of intrascrotal swelling.

PERI-ORCHITIS

This presents as a tender nodule on the surface of the testis and results from inflammation in the tunica vaginalis. Symptoms usually improve with time without the need for surgery.

CREMASTERIC SPASM

This may cause pain or discomfort, particularly during intercourse, and is associated with the testis being drawn up to the external inguinal ring. This may be relieved by circumcision of the cremaster which divides the genitofemoral nerve.

EPIDIDYMAL CYSTS

These are common and usually painless. Pain or discomfort may result from bleeding within a cyst. Referral is not required for asymptomatic cysts.

AFTER VASECTOMY

Scrotal discomfort after vasectomy may be caused by obstruction and distension of the epididymal duct. This is usually relieved by using a scrotal support and treatment with NSAIDs.

A small, tender swelling at the site of the vasectomy is frequently a sperm granuloma and may appear months or years after the procedure. If the pain fails to settle with a scrotal support and NSAIDs a surgical excision or epididymectomy may be required.

VARICOCELE

Varicoceles may cause aching within the scrotum which becomes worse towards the end of the day. Thrombosis within a varicocele has been reported as a cause of scrotal pain.

IDIOPATHIC

In many young men with scrotal pain the only abnormality found is a rather sensitive epididymis. This may result from 'seminal congestion' and is best treated by reassurance.

Important management points

1. Consider referral to GU medicine if you think there is evidence of epididymitis.
2. Consider urgent referral to Urology if there is a possibility of torsion.
3. Scrotal ultrasound is a useful non-invasive procedure that may help to determine the nature of intrascrotal pathology.

CHAPTER 16

Penile rashes

Inflammation of the glans penis (balanitis) and of the prepuce (posthitis) usually occur together.

IRRITANT BALANOPOSTHITIS

Very common and usually the result of poor hygiene. An accumulation of smegma may be visible. Advise gentle bathing twice daily with plain or slightly salty water followed by application of a barrier cream (e.g. aqueous cream).

CANDIDIASIS

Usually presents as a diffuse erythema with numerous scattered small, red, slightly 'eroded' spots (Plate 16.1).

BACTERIAL INFECTION

Anaerobic bacteria and group B streptococci occasionally cause a balano-posthitis. In the early stages of infection, gentle bathing followed by a barrier cream may be sufficient treatment.

DERMATITIS

Seborrhoeic dermatitis and contact dermatitis may present on the penis. Ask about other skin problems (e.g. affecting the scalp or face) and whether there is a history of allergy. Treat initially with hydrocortisone cream. If there is secondary infection consider using a combined steroidal/antibac-terial/antifungal preparation.

Less common causes of balanoposthitis include:

CIRCINATE BALANITIS

Associated with Reiter's syndrome or, more frequently, with the incomplete syndrome (i.e. reactive arthritis with or without urethritis or conjunctivitis: Plate 16.2).

LICHEN PLANUS

Usually presents with well-demarcated red-purplish lesions and may be confused with flat warts or psoriasis (Plate 16.3).

EARLY HUMAN PAPILLOMAVIRUS INFECTION

A patchy balanoposthitis may predate the appearance of classical condylomata acuminata (genital warts).

PSORIASIS

Genital lesions frequently lose the classical silvery scale and present as erythematous plaques.

LICHEN SCLEROSUS ET ATROPHICUS

Areas of erythema with whitened, atrophic patches are the typical features (Plate 16.4). Adhesions may occur between the glans penis and the prepuce and long-standing cases may progress to phimosis. Perimeatal disease leads to narrowing of the urethral meatus. Treat initially with a potent topical steroid (e.g. clobetasol propionate) and then slowly 'wean down' according to clinical response. Long-term follow-up is recommended because of the small risk of developing squamous cell carcinoma.

FIXED DRUG ERUPTIONS

Although many drugs have the potential to cause a fixed drug eruption it is more commonly seen with tetracyclines, sulphonamides, penicillin and salicylates. Lesions may first appear as a patch of erythema or a small blister and can rapidly progress to produce large areas of ulceration (Plate 16.5). Secondary infection can occur and treatment should include gentle bathing with salty water and, in some cases, a mild anti-inflammatory plus antibacterial cream. Oral prednisolone is very occasionally required for the more severe and extensive cases.

ZOON'S BALANITIS (PLASMA CELL BALANITIS)

An uncommon condition seen mostly in middle-aged and elderly men. The lesions present as flat, moist, red, shiny plaques affecting the glans and mucosa of the prepuce (Plate 16.6). Irritation is common. Although circumcision is a recommended treatment, some cases do respond to aeration and topical moderate-strength steroids.

ERYTHROPLASIA OF QUEYRAT

A very uncommon condition seen almost exclusively in uncircumcised men. Lesions appear as well-demarcated shiny, red, velvety plaques. Malignant change is common.

OTHER PENILE AND SCROTAL RASHES

Kaposi's sarcoma

Kaposi's sarcoma is seen mostly in patients with HIV infection in the U.K. and a number of studies have suggested that a herpes virus may be the causative agent. Lesions are initially flat and dusky red and may appear on the glans penis or shaft.

Angiokeratomata

These small lesions usually affect the scrotum rather than the penis and appear as tiny, often multiple, bright red vascular spots. They may increase in number and size with age and are harmless.

Melanocytic naevi

These may appear on the penis or scrotum and have the same characteristics as naevi elsewhere on the body.

General advice for patients with balanoposthitis

Aeration is helpful for most causes of balanitis but can sometimes be difficult to achieve. Keeping the foreskin retracted for an hour or so each evening and allowing a good circulation of air, perhaps under a dressing gown or nightshirt for social acceptability, is worth trying. A topical steroid or antibacterial cream, if indicated, can then be applied and the foreskin pulled back over the glans. It is unnecessary to use large amounts of cream and patients should be advised accordingly.

Gentle bathing with salty water is often soothing, particularly for moist lesions. The area can then be dried with a hair dryer on cool setting.

CHAPTER 17

Genital ulceration

Genital herpes

Herpes simplex virus (HSV) infection is by far the commonest cause of genital ulceration seen in general practice. Although HSV type 2 has traditionally been considered the commonest cause of genital herpes, recent studies have reported HSV type 1 infection in over 60% of cases, the virus being passed on by orogenital contact.

Serological studies examining HSV-2 seroprevalence in various population groups have shown that up to 70% of infections are asymptomatic.

Clinical features

PRIMARY ATTACK (i.e. NO PREVIOUS EXPOSURE TO HSV-1 OR HSV-2)

Primary herpes is a miserable condition. Following an incubation period of 3–5 days (range 1–40 days) small blisters appear on the genitalia, often associated with a 'flu-like' illness. The blisters soon break down to leave small tender ulcers that may eventually merge to produce quite extensive areas of painful ulceration (Figs 17.1 and 17.2). Lesions start to heal after about 12 days.

Herpes may cause a urethritis which presents as dysuria, often severe in nature.

Ninety per cent of women have a cervicitis producing an excessive 'vaginal' discharge.

Other clinical features include painful inguinal lymphadenopathy, headache and photophobia (aseptic meningitis), urinary retention (sacral radiculopathy), pharyngitis and extragenital lesions (finger, lip, buttock).

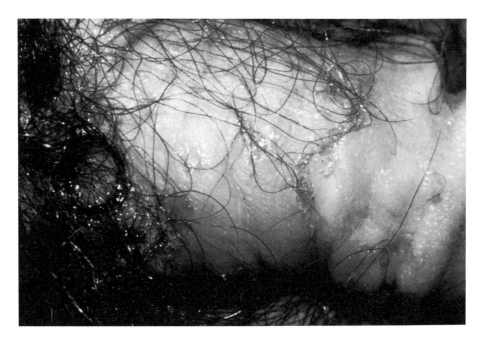

Fig. 17.1 Primary genital herpes affecting the penis.

FIRST ATTACK: NON-PRIMARY

This is the first clinical episode of herpes in a patient who has had previous exposure to the virus (type 1 or type 2). Symptoms are usually much less severe than primary herpes owing to partial immunity.

RECURRENT HERPES

Approximately 90% of patients with type 2 genital herpes will suffer a recurrence within 1 year of their primary attack. This is in contrast to patients with HSV type 1 infection, in whom there is a 55% chance of recurrence. The frequency of recurrences also differs between the two viral types – on average 3–4 attacks per year with HSV-2 infection compared with twice a year with HSV-1.

Viral reactivation leading to symptomatic or asymptomatic viral shedding may be greatest during the first few months after a primary attack and should be discussed with patients diagnosed with primary infection. Symptoms of recurrent genital herpes are often mild. About 50% of patients will develop prodromal symptoms such as genital 'pins and needles', shooting pains in the buttocks and legs or inguinal discomfort associated

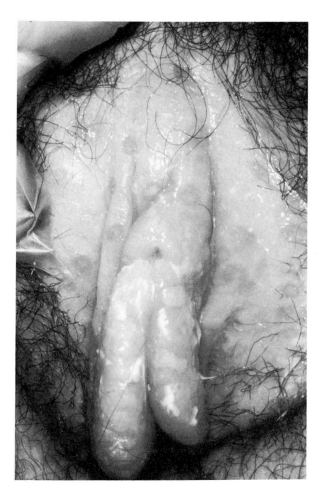

Fig. 17.2 Primary genital herpes affecting the vulva.

with lymphadenopathy. Symptoms of sacral neuralgia are the most trouble-some part of the recurrence for some patients.

The cervix is affected in only 10% of women with recurrent disease.

When lesions appear they tend to be few in number and heal within one week. A small number of patients, however, suffer more frequent and long-lasting attacks that can be particularly distressing (Figs 17.3 and 17.4).

Recent studies have suggested that symptoms of recurrent disease may be minimal and often ignored by the patient. This is an important issue that should be addressed when the diagnosis of herpes is first made. Taking note of minor genital symptoms and avoiding sexual contact at such times is important if the risk of transmission to partners is to be reduced.

It is always wise to confirm the clinical diagnosis of herpes by positive

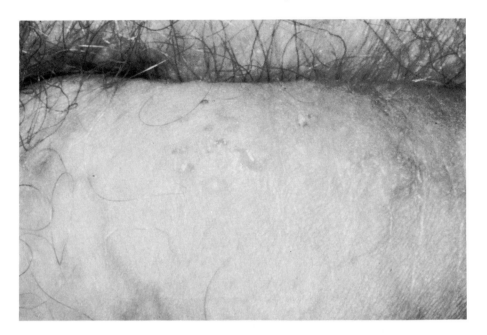

Fig. 17.3 Recurrent genital herpes affecting the penis. Vesicles, ulcers and scabbed lesions are visible.

viral culture. This may require patients re-attending immediately new genital sores appear so that further swabs can be taken for herpes culture.

Diagnosis of genital herpes

CULTURE

Many laboratories are now able to perform herpes typing. This is of some prognostic significance regarding recurrence rate (see above) and can be helpful information when counselling patients.

The chances of obtaining a positive culture will depend very much on the stage of the lesion: ulcers shed more virus than crusting lesions. This needs to be explained to the patient who may not fully appreciate why they were diagnosed as having herpes at their initial consultation and then told a week or two later that their 'herpes test' was negative. Herpes serology is currently of no diagnostic value. Serological assays which distinguish between HSV type 1 and type 2 antibodies are only available in a small number of research laboratories worldwide.

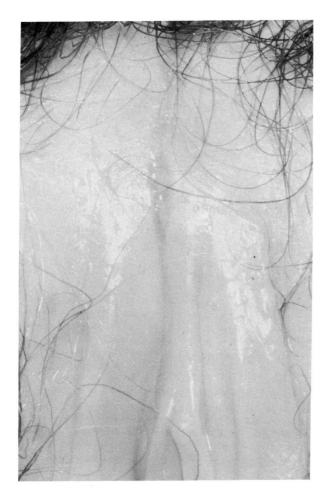

Fig. 17.4 Recurrent genital herpes affecting the vulva. It may be misdiagnosed as candidiasis.

Management

PRIMARY GENITAL HERPES

Women tend to fare rather worse than men. The genital sores are often exquisitely tender, urination may be intolerable and patients usually feel generally very unwell with myalgia, headaches, fever, etc. Recommendations:

— Take a swab for herpes virus culture.
— Aspirin or paracetamol (or stronger preparation) as required.

- Bathe the genital area twice daily with warm salty water and dry with the hair dryer on cool setting.
- Some women find it easier to pass urine while sitting in a warm bath.
- Aciclovir tablets 200 mg five times a day for 5 days, famciclovir 250 mg tds for 5 days or valaciclovir 500 mg bd for 5 days.
- There is no place for topical aciclovir cream in treating primary herpes.

Urinary retention secondary to sacral radiculopathy is uncommon and affects women and homosexual men more commonly than heterosexual men. Carbachol may prevent the need for catheterisation.

Approximately 10% of women suffer coincidental vaginal candidiasis. If there is generalised vulval erythema in addition to areas of ulceration or if symptoms persist after the ulcers have healed consider treating for *Candida* with an oral agent such as fluconazole 150 mg stat dose or itraconazole 200 mg bd for 1 day. Most women are rather too sore to use pessaries or cream.

The diagnosis of herpes can be psychologically traumatic and a great deal of time is often required to provide adequate information about the disease. Some patients require further more intensive 'counselling' to help them come to terms with the condition. Key issues which need to be addressed include the possibility of asymptomatic viral shedding, the effect this may have on current or future sexual relationships and the use of condoms to provide some protection to sexual partners. The issue of herpes in pregnancy is discussed below.

RECURRENT HERPES

Most patients cope extremely well with herpes. Attacks are usually infrequent and last only a few days and can be managed quite adequately by bathing the affected area with salty water and avoiding sexual contact while lesions are present.

A small number of patients suffer rather more painful and prolonged attacks and may benefit from a course of famciclovir (125 mg bd for 5 days), aciclovir tablets (200 mg five times a day for 3–5 days) or aciclovir cream (which must be used five times a day) taken or applied immediately lesions appear. There is currently some debate regarding the treatment of recurrent herpes with intermittent short courses of antiviral agents and concern has been raised about the possibility of generating resistant viral strains. It is therefore worth emphasising that most patients with recurrent herpes do not require therapy.

For the small minority of patients who are plagued by very frequent and prolonged recurrences it may be worth considering prophylactic aciclovir. This entails taking tablets on a daily basis for up to 1 year initially after which time the medication is stopped and the frequency of recurrences re-assessed. Patients may be started on 200 mg four times a day and reviewed at 3-monthly intervals, the dosage being reduced to a level that will prevent recurrences. Some patients can be maintained on a tds or, very occasionally, a bd dosage. An alternative approach is to prescribe 400 mg bd from the outset.

PREGNANCY

Neonatal herpes carries a significant mortality and morbidity but is fortunately a rare condition in this country. The baby is at greatest risk if the mother develops primary herpes during the last trimester, particularly towards the time of labour. Interestingly, recent studies have shown that most babies with neonatal herpes acquire their infection from mothers with asymptomatic primary herpes who are shedding virus during the birth.

There is minimal risk to the baby in women with recurrent disease. This is probably related to protective antibody passing across the placenta and to a much lower rate of viral shedding from the cervix in recurrent disease compared with primary infection. This is important to mention after diagnosing herpes as issues regarding future pregnancies are high on the list of worries. Women with a past history of genital herpes should be advised to present early in labour and undergo a careful examination for evidence of genital lesions. Although there is minimal risk to the baby, in view of the severity of neonatal herpes most obstetricians would advise caesarean section rather than vaginal delivery if lesions are present.

The diagnosis and management of genital herpes can sometimes pose problems. Referral to GU medicine should therefore be considered even if just for discussion and to provide information.

Other causes of genital ulceration

CANDIDIASIS

Vulval candidiasis may occasionally be mistaken for genital herpes particularly when there is severe vulval soreness with disruption of the vulva epithelium. Conversely, recurrent herpes may produce only minor vulval discomfort and be dismissed by the patient as simply an attack of 'thrush'.

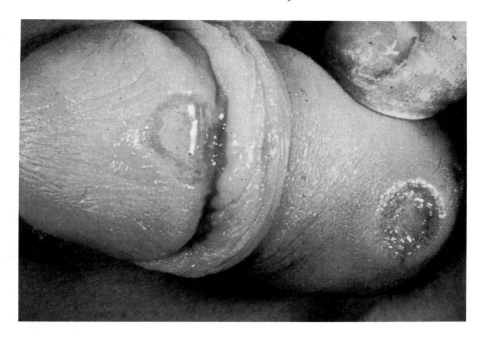

Fig. 17.5 Chancres of primary syphilis.

For this reason it is important to explain to patients with a history of herpes that minor genital symptoms may be a recurrence of their herpes and that necessary care should be taken during sexual intercourse.

SYPHILIS

Although textbooks quite correctly mention syphilis in the differential diagnosis of genital ulceration, this is now fortunately a rare disease in the U.K. The primary chancre of primary syphilis is usually painless, although secondary infection may produce some tenderness (Fig. 17.5). Patients should be referred to GU medicine if there is the slightest doubt regarding the clinical diagnosis of genital ulceration. Dark-ground microscopy for treponemes can be performed on site and optimal specimens will be obtained for herpes culture. Remember that syphilis serology is usually negative in primary syphilis and may not become positive for up to 3 months after infection. For this reason, all patients should have syphilis serology performed at 3 months after presentation if the cause of genital ulceration is uncertain.

FIXED DRUG ERUPTION

More severe cases may lead to ulceration (see p. 65).

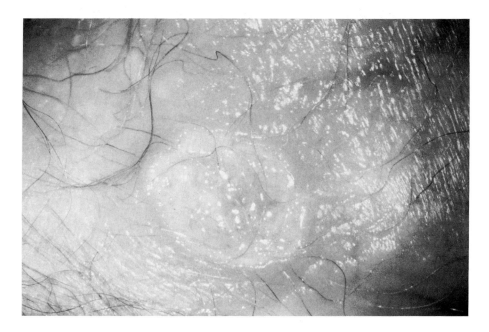

Fig. 17.6 Behçet's disease. Typical scrotal ulcer.

CHANCROID AND LYMPHOGRANULOMA VENEREUM

These are common tropical STDs but rare in the U.K. Remember to ask about sexual contact when abroad.

BEHÇET'S DISEASE

The genital ulcers in this condition are tender and usually have a well-demarcated edge (Fig. 17.6). To make a diagnosis of Behçet's disease there should also be a history of oral ulceration together with eye, skin or neurological complications.

In women, one more commonly sees simple aphthous ulceration affecting the mouth and labia, there being no other features to suggest Behçet's disease.

ULCERS OF LIPSCHUTZ

In 1913, Lipschutz described cases of acute vulval ulceration associated with fever and lymphadenopathy. More recently, genital ulceration has been described as an uncommon complication of infectious mononucleosis and it is therefore possible that Lipschutz's original cases related to Epstein–Barr virus infection.

BULLOUS SKIN CONDITIONS

Pemphigus and cicatricial pemphigoid very occasionally present on the genitalia. The bullae may be short-lived leaving areas of eroded epithelium.

> Any case of genital ulceration for which a definitive diagnosis cannot be made should ideally be referred to GU medicine for assessment and further investigation.

CHAPTER 18

Genital 'lumps'

Genital warts

The most frequently seen genital 'lumps' in general practice are genital warts or condylomata acuminata ('pointed condylomata'). The term 've-nereal warts' is now outdated and should not be used. Genital warts are the second commonest STD in the U.K. and are caused by human papilloma (HPV), which is the commonest sexually transmitted viral infection in the U.K. Recent studies using an extremely sensitive method of detecting HPV DNA (polymerase chain reaction) suggest that many sexually active people carry low levels of HPV in the genital tract but only a small number of infected individuals develop warts. The natural history and infectivity of this so-called 'subclinical' HPV infection is unknown.

MANAGEMENT OF GENITAL WARTS

Patients with genital warts should ideally be referred to GU medicine for assessment and initiation of treatment, irrespective of the age of the patient and the length of time the warts have been present. Genital warts are almost always sexually acquired (Figs 18.1 and 18.2), although lesions may have been present for many months or even years before the patient seeks a medical opinion. Very occasionally hand warts may be transferred to the genitalia and this should be considered if the lesions resemble planar warts rather than condylomata acuminata.

The incubation period between acquiring HPV infection and the appearance of warts may be many months, which can lead to some difficulty in determining exactly when and from whom the infection was caught.

Anal warts (Fig. 18.3) are commonly seen in both women and heterosexual men, either with or without genital lesions, and these may extend into the anal canal. Anal warts are not indicative of anal intercourse; the

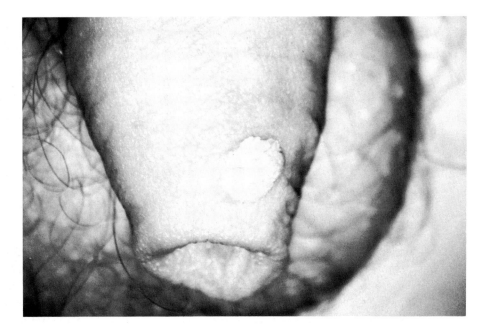

Fig. 18.1 Genital wart (condylomata acuminata) affecting the penile shaft.

method by which HPV is transferred to the anus of a heterosexual male is currently unknown.

HPV infection is sexually acquired and most patients should be checked for other STDs, in particular chlamydial infection. Remember that STDs are frequently carried without symptoms. Sexual partners should be carefully assessed, which for female partners should include vaginal and cervical examination, ideally with a colposcope.

TREATMENT

(1) Cryotherapy is an extremely effective and generally well-tolerated treatment that does not require a local anaesthetic. This is a useful first-line treatment.

(2) Podophyllin is a time-honoured treatment that requires application by medical staff twice or thrice weekly. The patient should wash off the paint after 4–6 h as prolonged application can lead to burning and ulceration. Fresh, moist warts may respond well to this form of treatment. Once keratin has started to appear on the wart surface success is less likely.

(3) Podophyllotoxin is a pure preparation of one of the active ingredients

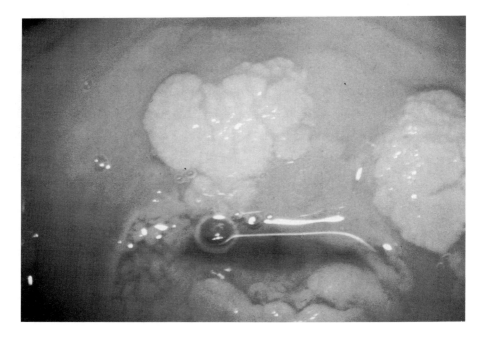

Fig. 18.2 Cervical warts.

of podophyllin and has the advantage of self-application. It is quite expensive compared with podophyllin but is highly effective in patients with fresh lesions and is ideal for those who find it difficult to adhere to regular clinic or surgery attendance. Some women find it difficult to apply, particularly if lesions are small, and treatment of anal warts usually requires some assistance.

(4) Trichloracetic acid acts as a caustic agent and can be useful for burning off small warts. To be used with care!

(5) Diathermy, scissor excision and laser ablation require a local anaesthetic; prior application of prilocaine plus lignocaine cream makes this more tolerable. Very useful for persistent warts and should be considered earlier rather than later in the course of treatment.

OTHER MANAGEMENT ISSUES

Genital warts have a tendency to recur, in some cases with alarming frequency. Such patients may require psychological support.

Most clinicians advise the use of condoms while warts are present. Although HPV remains in the epithelium after warts have cleared, the degree of infectivity of subclinically carried virus is currently unknown.

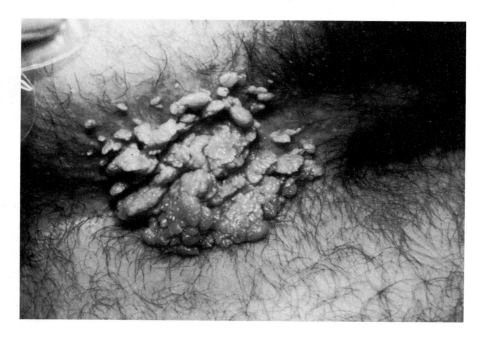

Fig. 18.3 Anal warts.

It is therefore very difficult to accurately advise for how long condoms should be used after apparently successful treatment.

HPV INFECTION AND ANOGENITAL CANCER

There is now a good deal of evidence linking HPV infection with cervical, vulval, penile and anal squamous cell carcinoma. Most studies have focused on cervical neoplasia and dysplasia (or CIN; Plates 18.1 and 18.2) and have shown certain HPV types to have a greater potential to induce dysplastic and neoplastic change. The commonest so-called 'high risk' types are HPV-16 and 18. HPV-6 and 11 are found in genital warts and are considered 'low-risk' HPV types. As mentioned earlier, many sexually active people harbour low levels of HPV in the genital tract, including the high-risk types 16 or 18. In some individuals this infection eventually clears, in others it may persist indefinitely but pose no problem. In a small number of individuals, HPV infection may induce cellular dysplastic change. Dysplasia may revert to normal over time or, again in a small number of individuals, progress to neoplastic change. The chances of an individual infected with a 'high-risk' HPV type developing a cervical cancer depends on several factors. These include the quantity of virus present, the genetically deter-

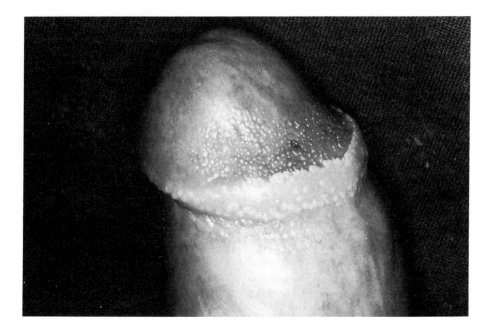

Fig. 18.4 Hirsutes papillaris penis.

mined immunological host response to the virus and other cofactors such as smoking, herpes simplex virus coinfection and possibly the presence of other genital infections.

Some clinicians believe that women with genital warts have an increased risk for developing cervical neoplasia and therefore advise annual cervical cytology. This is currently an issue for debate and awaits further study.

Other causes of genital 'lumps'

HIRSUTES PAPILLARIS PENIS

'Hirsutes papillaris penis' or 'penile pearly pink papules' is one of the commonest conditions to be mistaken for genital warts in men. The lesions appear as rows of small pink or white filiform papillae on the corona of the glans penis and by the frenulum (Fig. 18.4). They first appear at puberty and are found to varying degrees in up to 20% of men. They are harmless but a frequent cause of anxiety; if you are unsure, ask GU medicine to assess. Tiny papules by the frenulum can be difficult to distinguish from warts and may require examination with the aid of a magnifying glass or colposcope.

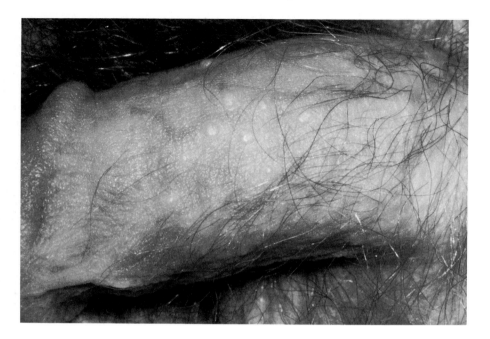

Fig. 18.5 Molluscum contagiosum.

Vulval micropapillae

Many women have small finger-like projections on the inner surface of the labia minora and around the introitus. These are benign micropapillae (Plate 18.3) and may be seen in conjunction with warts, which often makes clinical assessment quite difficult. The current consensus of opinion is that these micropapillae are not related to HPV infection and therefore do not warrant treatment. Examination with some form of magnification, such as the colposcope, is often required to differentiate these lesions from genital warts.

Fordyce spots

'Fordyce spots' (Plate 18.4) are commonly seen in both men and women. They are a normal variant, thought to be ectopic sebaceous glands, which appear as tiny cream coloured spots just under the skin surface.

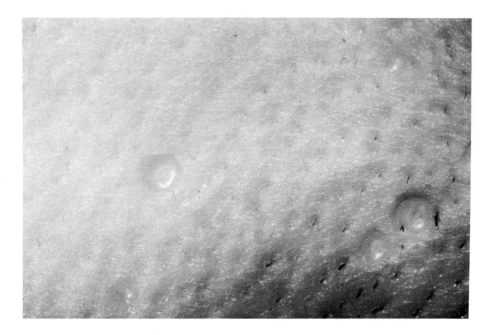

Fig. 18.6 Molluscum contagiosum.

Molluscum contagiosum

Lesions are classically smooth and rounded with a central punctum although polypoid forms are occasionally seen (Figs 18.5 and 18.6). Treatment is with cryotherapy. Applying phenol with a sharpened orange stick tends to be less well tolerated.

Sebaceous cysts

These present as round, creamy-yellow, smooth swellings. Scrotal cysts may reach a centimetre in diameter and are often multiple (Fig. 18.7).

Lichen planus

Papular lesions of lichen planus may be mistaken for flat or papular warts. Diagnosis is aided by the violaceous colour and the presence of fine white linear striae (Wickham's striae).

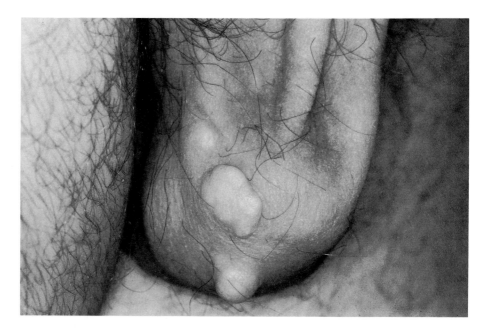

Fig. 18.7 Scrotal sebaceous cysts.

Lichen nitidus

An uncommon condition presenting as very tiny pink or brown, dome-shaped, shiny papules. They may be found in conjunction with lichen planus.

Psoriasis

Plaques of psoriasis may occasionally be misdiagnosed as flat warts. Genital lesions often lack the characteristic silvery scale leaving a red, slightly shiny surface.

Condylomata lata

A feature of secondary syphilis that present as pink or grey, moist, slightly elevated lesions (Plate 18.5). There are often other signs of syphilis (e.g. generalised rash, oral lesions, lymphadenopathy) and syphilis serology

(VDRL (Venereal Diseases Research Laboratories) and TPHA (*Treponema pallidum* haemagglutination assay)) will be positive at this stage of the disease.

Carcinoma

Neoplastic lesions usually feel hard or gritty, often bleed on contact and may be ulcerated. Genital warts rarely undergo malignant change but any suspicious lesion requires biopsy.

Lymphocele

A common condition presenting as a smooth, firm, worm-like cord in or below the coronal sulcus just below the glans penis. There may be a history of recent strenuous sexual activity. There is no specific treatment and the condition resolves with time.

Peyronie's disease

A condition of unknown cause characterised by the development of fibrous plaques within the penis. The first sign noted by the patient is often a painless lump, sometimes associated with discomfort on erection. As the condition progresses the penis may bend to one side on erection, occasionally making intercourse impossible. Many patients improve spontaneously with time (often months or years) and reassurance is usually all that is required. Potassium *para*-aminobenzoate (POTABA), vitamin E and intralesional triamcinolone injection have been tried, usually with little success. Surgery is best reserved for those patients with a penile deformity that interferes with intercourse.

CHAPTER 19

Genital irritation

The patient presenting with genital irritation should be asked:

– Exactly where is the irritation: penis, scrotum, towards the entrance of the vagina, on the labia majora, above the genitalia in the pubic area?
– Is there anything to see, such as a rash, warts or pubic lice?
– Is there irritation elsewhere on the body?

The commonest causes of genital irritation are:

– Dermatoses: dermatitis, lichen simplex, lichen planus, lichen sclerosus et atrophicus, etc.
– Infection: candidiasis, early genital herpes (preulcerative stage), HPV infection (warts or VIN (vulval intraepithelial neoplasia)), trichomoniasis, pubic lice.

These conditions are mostly covered in other sections (see Chapters 8 and 16). This chapter will focus on the two common parasitic infections: pubic lice and scabies.

Pubic lice ('crabs' or pediculosis)

The pubic louse (*Phthirus pubis*) may spread to any hairy part of the body with the exception of the scalp and eyebrows. Very occasionally the eyelashes may be involved. Transmission is by body contact although toilet seats and shared clothing have been implicated in a small number of cases. Pubic lice are very slow movers and live for only a day away from the host.

SYMPTOMS

Irritation is the commonest presenting symptom and the severity will depend on the level of hypersensitivity to mite antigen. In a previously unexposed individual symptoms may take up to 5 days to occur. Excessive scratching can sometimes lead to excoriation and secondary infection. A large infestation resulting in multiple bites over a short period of time may cause mild fever and general malaise.

SIGNS

A careful search for eggs (nits) and lice may be required in milder infections. To the uninitiated, lice resemble 'freckles' or small brown 'scabs'. Pubic lice move on average a maximum of only 10 cm a day so it is unusual to see any activity during a 6 min consultation.

MANAGEMENT

Clothing should be laundered in hot water or by dry cleaning.

The most widely used pediculosides are 1% lindane (gamma benzene hexachloride) lotion and 0.5% malathion lotion. The preparation should be rubbed into the hairs and washed off 12 h later. Although a second treatment is recommended after 1 week to kill any lice emerging from surviving eggs, the presence of eggs does not signify treatment failure. Lindane should be avoided during pregnancy or breast feeding, in young children and in patients with severely excoriated lesions because of the possibility of absorption leading to neurotoxicity.

The possibility of itching persisting after successful treatment should be mentioned to the patient. If this proves a problem consider using topical hydrocortisone or an oral antihistamine, such as one of the sedative preparations, at night.

Shaving the hair is unnecessary and may aggravate the irritation.

Sexual contacts should be assessed and treated as appropriate.

An infestation affecting the eye-lashes may be effectively treated by applying vaseline gently to the lashes.

Scabies

The scabies mite (*Sarcoptes scabei*) is much smaller than the pubic louse and is only just visible to the naked eye. Transmission is by close personal contact and occasionally by wearing infected clothes. Although scabies is seen in school-age children transmission within schools is uncommon. Outbreaks occasionally occur in nursing homes, hospitals and other institutions. The incubation period for a first attack is up to 8 weeks with subsequent attacks producing symptoms within a few days because of previous sensitisation.

SYMPTOMS

Irritation tends to be generalised, sparing the head, and is worse at night.

SIGNS

Genital lesions are generally found only in men and appear as nodules on the penile shaft and scrotum. There is usually evidence of scabies elsewhere, particularly favoured sites being the finger webs and sides of the fingers, flexor surfaces of the wrists, extensor surfaces of the elbows, anterior axillary folds, umbilicus, nipples and buttock creases.

Classical lesions include:

- short, wavy, dirty appearing burrows
- small, erythematous, eczematous papules
- small nodules (penis, scrotum).

The scalp, face and neck are spared in adults. Scratch marks are frequently seen and secondary eczematisation and infection may mask the other features and make diagnosis rather more difficult.

DIAGNOSIS

Scabies is often diagnosed purely on clinical grounds: intense irritation, especially at night, characteristic lesions, similar complaints in household members or sexual partners. Where possible, however, an attempt should be made to confirm the diagnosis which involves identifying the mite, eggs or larvae under the microscope. First place a drop or two of indian ink on to a suspected burrow and remove any excess with an alcohol wipe. This helps to 'highlight' the burrow which should then be scraped gently with a scalpel blade and the material obtained transferred to a microscope slide. Apply a coverslip and examine with a microscope using low-power magnification.

MANAGEMENT

1. All household members and sexual partners should be treated: they may remain asymptomatic for up to 8 weeks and during that time spread the disease unknowingly.

2. All patients should be warned to expect continued irritation for as long as 3 months after successful treatment.
3. Warn patients against overtreatment that can cause an irritant dermatitis.
4. Lotions are easier to apply than creams.
5. The lotion should be applied to all of the skin from the neck downwards with particular attention to palms, soles, interdigital spaces and genitals. This is most easily performed with a 3–5 cm paint brush and help is usually required to reach the more distant areas.
6. Bathing before the lotion is applied is unnecessary and may increase systemic absorption of the scabicide.
7. Re-infection from bedlinen and clothing is no longer considered a risk.

The treatment of choice is lindane (gamma benzene hexachloride, 1% lotion) which has a pleasant smell and can be used on eczematous skin. Leaving the preparation on for 6 h cures 96% of cases compared with a 98% cure rate if the preparation is left for 12–24 h. There is the possibility of neurotoxicity, so lindane is not recommended for children under 10 years of age, pregnant and breast feeding women.

Malathion is also a non-irritant scabicide and is applied as a 0.5% lotion or aqueous emulsion. The preparation should be washed off after 24 h.

Monosulfiram is dispensed as a 25% solution in industrial methylated spirit which needs to be diluted in two to three parts of water immediately before application. A single application may be as good as the recommended application on 2–3 consecutive nights. Patients should avoid alcohol for 2–3 days after treatment because of the possibility of a disulfiram-like reaction.

Troublesome post-treatment pruritis usually responds to an oral antihistamine or topical hydrocortisone.

CHAPTER 20

Human immunodeficiency virus (HIV) infection

GU medicine physicians provide most of the out-patient care, and in some hospitals also the in-patient care, for patients with HIV infection. The diagnosis still carries a certain stigma and may bring to the forefront emotions regarding sexuality or drug abuse. AIDS has received a tremendous amount of hype by 'medical' journalists and social commentators and although HIV is a devastating infection it should be viewed in the context of other life-threatening diseases. This chapter deals with just a few of the important issues regarding HIV antibody testing and patient management.

HIV antibody testing

1. Many people request an HIV antibody test for 'peace of mind'. They may be entering a new sexual relationship and wish to clear up a nagging doubt about a previous partner. It is important to try and assess the degree of risk: has there been previous sexual contact with bisexual or homosexual men, injecting drug users or persons from 'high-risk' areas of the world? Of course one can never be certain exactly what previous partners or their previous partners have been up to and so direct questioning only provides a rough guide to the true risk. Although an unexpected positive result occasionally turns up, more commonly there is a clue from the history. Remember that injecting users who deny ever sharing needles and syringes ('works') may have been exposed to HIV from their sexual partners who do share needles.

2. Following infection with HIV there is a delay of between 3 and 6 months before antibodies become detectable on serology. This 'window period' needs to be explained to the patient and testing possibly delayed until sufficient time has elapsed after potential exposure. For this reason testing is often performed at 3 months after exposure and then again at

6 months. Seroconversion after 6 months has been reported but is considered a rare event.

3. Although needle-stick injuries are more common in the hospital setting occasionally the GP will be consulted following an injury in the community or in the surgery. The risk of acquiring HIV from a needle-stick injury from an infected patient is approximately 0.3%. The risk of transmission following an injury from a needle of 'unknown origin' is obviously less. The risk of acquiring hepatitis B following a needle-stick injury from an 'e antigen' positive patient is 30% and the risk of hepatitis C infection from a needle-stick injury is approximately 3%. If the injury were sustained by a doctor or nurse from a patient in the surgery, direct questioning will help to determine the risk of infection, although bear in mind that questions regarding sexuality and drug use may not always be answered honestly and that some infected patients give no history of 'risk contact'. If there is concern, ask the patient whether they would consent to being tested for HIV, hepatitis B and, if intravenous drug misuse is suspected, hepatitis C infection. If consent is denied and there is a definite risk of infection, consider a booster dose of hepatitis B vaccine, assuming that the healthcare worker has been previously vaccinated and that antibody levels are unknown. HIV serology should be performed at 3 and 6 months and condoms used during this time.

   Specific hepatitis B immunoglobulin (HBIG) in addition to hepatitis B vaccination should be considered for patients sustaining a needle-stick injury in the community. A careful evaluation is required in each case to determine the true risk and whether prophylaxis is needed. If in doubt err on the side of caution. HBIG should be given preferably within 48 h and not later than a week after exposure at a dose of 200 IU for children 0–4 years, 300 IU for children 5–9 years and 500 IU for adults and children over 10 years. HIV serology should be performed at 3 and 6 months. Discussion with your local Public Health Laboratory is advisable; they may already have guidelines for the management of needle-stick injuries in general practice.

4. Insurance companies used to ask new clients to state whether they had previously had an HIV antibody test or considered themselves at potential risk of acquiring HIV whereas now most ask whether there has been a previous positive test for HIV. Having previously been tested negative for HIV should no longer cause difficulties when applying for life insurance.

5. Some 'HIV-workers' have suggested that HIV pretest counselling should only be performed by experienced counsellors within depart-

ments of GU medicine or specialised testing centres. This is a rather extreme view. There is no reason why HIV antibody testing should not be performed in general practice; however, there are a few points worth considering. Firstly, for reasons of confidentiality many patients prefer not to have a record of HIV antibody testing in their general practice notes. If the result proves positive then of course it is important that the general practitioner is aware of the diagnosis. Secondly, patients with possible risk factors for infection may be better assessed and tested in the GU medicine setting where full support can be provided if the result is positive. Thirdly, if an individual is concerned about possible sexual exposure to HIV then it is wise to check for other sexually transmitted infections, such as *Chlamydia*, which are far more common than HIV.

6. Many GU medicine clinics now run 'fast service' HIV antibody testing that provides results within 24 h. This is ideal for the anxious patient who is deterred from testing because of a several day wait for results.

Clinical features and management

SEROCONVERSION ILLNESS

Over 50% of patients report a 'flu-like' or 'glandular-fever like' illness at the time of seroconversion (i.e. about 2–6 months after infection).

PERSISTENT GENERALISED LYMPHADENOPATHY

After a variable period of time a number of patients develop cervical and axillary lymphadenopathy. This is usually painless and the glands affected are usually > 1 cm diameter. Lymphadenopathy is of no prognostic significance.

CONSTITUTIONAL SYMPTOMS (PREVIOUSLY CALLED 'AIDS-RELATED COMPLEX' OR ARC)

Most patients with HIV remain asymptomatic for a number of years. During this time the virus is replicating in the lymphoid tissue and although the CD4 or T-helper lymphocytes are being destroyed, the immune system is sufficiently robust to maintain normal lymphocyte levels. After a period of usually some years, the immune system shows signs of deterioration and the CD4 lymphocyte count falls. This is sometimes associated with the development of constitutional symptoms (previously termed 'AIDS-related complex') such as loss of weight, night sweats, diarrhoea and profound lethargy. It is important to remember, however, that many patients with low CD4 cell counts are asymptomatic. Symptoms of constitutional HIV disease often improve with antiretroviral medication (e.g. zidovudine, didanosine, zalcitabine).

AIDS (ACQUIRED IMMUNODEFICIENCY SYNDROME)

This is an emotive and not particularly helpful term clinically. A diagnosis of AIDS signifies 'end-stage' HIV disease, although the prognosis even at this stage varies greatly according to the AIDS-defining diagnosis. Long-term prognosis, however, is generally poor with over 80% of patients dying within 3 years of the diagnosis of AIDS. Recent studies suggest that the mean period of time from acquiring HIV to the development of AIDS is 11 years. A small subgroup of patients with HIV remain clinically well for many years, which is probably the result of infection with a less virulent strain of virus. AIDS-defining conditions are listed in Table 20.1.

IMPORTANT MANAGEMENT POINTS

1. Clinical review every 3–6 months is advisable. When patients are well the fewer visits to the clinic the better as it often serves as an unhappy reminder of their diagnosis. A great deal of psychological support, however, may be required for the patient and, in many cases, sexual partners and the immediate family. This is particularly important at the time of diagnosis and during the early months after diagnosis.
2. Issues which should be addressed and discussed include:
   (a) Need to notify sexual or 'works-sharing' partners
   This is an important issue that requires careful discussion. Partner notification is one of the many tasks performed by the GU medicine clinic health adviser and should be considered when a patient is reluctant to contact a previous partner directly. Most patients, however, fully appreciate the need to inform previous contacts and take on this responsibility.
   (b) How to avoid passing on the infection (i.e. what sexual practices are safe or unsafe; safe-injecting practices)
   Condoms provide an adequate barrier to HIV; however, problems arise when they are not used consistently or when they split or slip off the penis. Extra strong condoms are available for anal intercourse, although these may occasionally tear, and remember to

Table 20.1. *AIDS Defining Conditions (1993 classification)*

Bacterial pneumonia (recurrent)
Candidiasis (oesophageal, tracheal or bronchial; not oral)
Cervical cancer (carcinoma *in situ* is not included)
Coccidiomycosis (disseminated or extrapulmonary)
Cryptococcal meningitis and other extrapulmonary disease
Cryptosporidiosis with diarrhoea persisting for >1 month
Cytomegalovirus disease (other than liver, spleen or lymph nodes)
Herpes simplex infection: ulceration persisting for longer than one month,
   bronchitis, pneumonitis, oesophagitis
HIV encephalopathy
HIV wasting syndrome
Histoplasmosis (disseminated or extrapulmonary)
Isosporiasis with diarrhoea persisting for >1 month
Kaposi's sarcoma
Lymphoma of the brain
Non-Hodgkin's lymphoma
Mycobacterium avium complex disease
Mycobacterium tuberculosis: any site (pulmonary or extrapulmonary)
Mycobacterium of other species: disseminated or extrapulmonary
Pneumocystis carinii pneumonia (PCP)
Progressive multifocal leucoencephalopathy
Salmonella septicaemia (recurrent)
Toxoplasmosis of the brain

HIV, human immunodeficiency virus.

advise the use of water-based rather than oil-based lubricants (see
Chapter 12).
   There is a small but definite risk of transmitting HIV through
oral sex: advise the use of a dental dam (a thin latex square) or
flavoured condoms.
   Practices which may draw blood, such as biting or scratching,
should be avoided.
   Kissing, mutual masturbation, body-rubbing are considered safe.
Injecting drug users should avoid sharing contaminated needles,
spoons and syringes ('works') and many pharmacists and drug agen-
cies now run needle-exchange schemes. Boiling used syringes and
needles is a less safe alternative. Flushing 'works' with bleach
reduces levels of active virus but is unreliable and should only be

considered when there is no reasonable alternative. Full-strength household bleach is required with a minimum contact time of 30 s.

(c) Who should be informed or needs to know the diagnosis

Advise the patient to think carefully before telling others of the diagnosis. Employers and work colleagues rarely need to be informed.

(d) Healthy lifestyle

This involves getting enough rest, taking exercise as tolerated, reducing and eventually stopping smoking, eating a 'healthy' diet and reducing unnecessary stress. Some patients benefit from complementary medical care such as reflexology, aromatherapy, facial massage and relaxation and visualisation techniques.

(e) Pregnancy and the risk to the infant

Most mother to baby transmission occurs late in pregnancy or during delivery. Transmission rates vary from 15 to 20% in Europe and are higher, in the region of 30%, in Africa. Recent studies have suggested that caesarean section and the use of zidovudine during pregnancy, delivery and the neonatal period will reduce the risk of transmission. The use of vaginal lavage with antiseptics and/or virucidal agents during labour is currently under study. Breast feeding carries an additional risk of transmission and should be advised against where there are safe alternatives. Breast feeding, however, is still recommended in the developing world where the protection against infectious disease outweighs the risk of HIV transmission.

(f) What support is available

Support will be available at both local and national level. Information about local support groups is best obtained from your local GU medicine clinic. A list of useful support services is provided at the end of the chapter.

(g) Immunisation

BCG and yellow fever vaccination should be avoided. Live attenuated vaccines for measles, mumps, rubella and polio may be given although it should be noted that polio virus may be excreted for longer periods than in uninfected persons.

Although pneumococcal vaccination has been recommended for HIV-positive patients, clinical efficacy has not been proven.

Further information on vaccination may be obtained from the HMSO publication *Immunisation against Infectious Disease*.

(h) Clinical follow-up

The importance of clinical follow-up should be stressed and an emphasis placed on the role of drugs to prevent complications and slow disease progression.

3. Baseline investigations performed routinely after diagnosis include:
   – Confirmatory HIV antibody test
   – Full blood count
   – T lymphocyte subsets (CD4 and CD8)
   – Liver function tests
   – Hepatitis B and C serology
   – Syphilis serology
   – *Toxoplasma* serology
   – Cytomegalovirus serology
   – Chest radiograph
   – Weight

4. The CD4 lymphocyte count should be measured on a regular basis as this provides some guide to immune status. The risk of developing *Pneumocystis carinii* pneumonia increases once the CD4 count falls below $200/mm^3$ and prophylaxis is recommended at this stage (e.g. co-trimoxazole 960 mg orally three times a week).

   Some clinicians would also recommend prophylaxis against oral and oesophageal candidiasis with oral antifungals (e.g. fluconazole 150 mg weekly), but recent studies suggest that this may lead to the development of drug resistance and so treating symptoms as they occur may be more appropriate. Nystatin pastilles or suspension or amphotericin lozenges are often effective for oral candidiasis.

5. Zidovudine improves the symptoms of constitutional disease in some patients and has been shown to prolong survival and reduce the risk of opportunistic infections in patients with AIDS and constitutional disease. The role of antiretrovirals in the management of patients with asymptomatic disease remains controversial.

6. Combination therapy with drugs acting at various stages of the HIV replicative cycle may prove to be the most effective approach to treatment. This could involve concurrent or sequential use of nucleoside analogue reverse transcriptase inhibitors (e.g. zidovudine, didanosine, zalcitabine, lamivudine), non-nucleoside analogue reverse transcriptase inhibitors (e.g. nevirapine) and protease inhibitors (e.g. saquinavir).

7. The 'shared-care' approach with general practitioners involved in clinical management along with the hospital team is a useful model that works extremely well in many districts. A multidisciplinary team is often required with hospital doctors, GPs, social workers, counsellors, dietitians, drug-workers and district nurses working closely together. Most teams also have a designated 'HIV liaison nurse' who plays

a key role in coordinating care and oversees the smooth transition between hospital and the community.

Management of the common complications of HIV infection are summarised in Table 20.2.

Table 20.2. *Common complications of HIV infection*

Symptoms	Common cause	Common treatment
Sore mouth ± dysphagia	*Candida* (Plate 20.1)	Nystatin pastilles or suspension; amphotericin lozenges; fluconazole; itraconazole
	Herpes simplex	Aciclovir; famciclovir; valaciclovir
Diarrhoea ± weight loss	*Cryptosporidium*	Codeine phosphate; loperamide; paromomycin
	HIV enteropathy	Codeine phosphate; loperamide
Headache	Cryptococcal meningitis	Amphotericin ± flucytosine; fluconazole
	Toxoplasmosis	Pyrimethamine + sulphadiazine/clindamycin
	Lymphoma	Prognosis very poor
Cough ± breathlessness	*Pneumocystis carinii*	Co-trimoxazole; pentamidine
	Bacterial pneumonia	Conventional therapy
Loss of vision	Cytomegalovirus retinitis	Ganciclovir; foscarnet
Fever/weight loss	*Mycobacterium avium* complex	Combination therapy, e.g. rifabutin, clofazimine, clarithromycin, ciprofloxacin
	Cytomegalovirus	Ganciclovir, foscarnet
	Non-Hodgkin's lymphoma	Chemotherapy, e.g. CHOP

Table 20.2. (*cont.*)

Other problems	Common treatment
Thrombocytopenia	Zidovudine; prednisolone (treatment often not required)
Kaposi's sarcoma (Plate 20.2)	Radiotherapy; vinblastine + bleomycin; liposomal doxorubicin; 'skin camouflage'
Herpes	Aciclovir; famciclovir; valaciclovir
Genital warts	Cryotherapy
Mollusum contagiosum	Cryotherapy
Seborrhoeic dermatitis	Antifungal + hydrocortisone cream

CHOP: cyclophosphamide, hydroxydaunorubicin, vincristine and prednisolone.

Support services and useful contacts in the U.K.

National AIDS Helpline
Tel: 0800 567123 (Free phone 24 h)

Gay Men Fighting AIDS
Tel: 0171 738 6872

Terrence Higgins Trust
52–54 Grays Inn Road, London WC1X 8JU
Tel: 0171 242 1010 (12 noon–10 pm)

Body Positive (London)
51b Philbeach Gardens, London SW5 9EB
Tel: 0171 835 1045
(There are Body Positive groups throughout the country. Information may be obtained from the London office.)

Positively Women
5 Sebastian Street, London EC1V 0HE
Tel: 0171 490 5515

BHAN (Black HIV/AIDS Network)
111 Devonport Road, London W12 8PB
Tel: 0181 742 9223

Blackliners
The Eurolink Centre, 49 Effra Road, London SW2 1BZ
Tel: 0171 738 5274

The Naz Project (Southern Asian and Muslim)
Palingswick House, 241 King Street, London W6 9LP
Tel: 0181 563 0191

Haemophilia Society
123 Westminster Bridge Road, London SE1 7HR
Tel: 0171 928 2020

Mainliners (Injecting drug users)
205 Stockwell Road, London SW9 9SL
Tel: 0171 738 4656

Positively Children
Jan Rebane Centre, 12–14 Thornton Street, London SW9 0BL
Tel: 0171 738 7333

Immunity Legal Centre
260a Kilburn Lane, London W10 4BA
Tel: 0181 968 8909
(Free legal advice for people in the London area infected with HIV.)

Scottish AIDS Monitor
26 Anderson Place, Edinburgh EH6 5NP
Tel: 0131 555 4850

CHAPTER 21

Genital problems in children

Paediatrics is usually the most appropriate first line of referral for children with genital problems requiring a specialist opinion. Referral on to gynaecology, urology, dermatology or GU medicine for a combined assessment can then take place if considered necessary. Consider seeking advice at an early stage, particularly if there is the slightest concern about sexual abuse. A telephone call and discussion prior to referral is often appreciated in the less straightforward cases.

Girls

VAGINAL DISCHARGE

Prepubertal girls do occasionally produce a small amount of clear, non-malodorous vaginal discharge. In addition, a slightly thicker, off-white discharge is often seen during the first week after birth and during the months preceding the menarche. A discharge which is particularly heavy or malodorous suggests an infective or pathological cause. This may be associated with vulval irritation and possibly evidence of vulval and vaginal erythema.

The more common causes of pathological discharge include:

1. Infection
   (a) Candidiasis
       As with adult infection, there is usually vulval irritation and evidence of a vulvitis. *Candida* may develop on a pre-existing skin disorder such as eczema or seborrhoeic dermatitis. It is worth enquiring whether the mother has symptoms suggestive of 'thrush' as transfer of *Candida* from mother to baby may sometimes occur.
   (b) Bacterial vaginosis
       Although usually associated with sexual activity, bacterial vaginosis

has been documented in sexually inexperienced adolescents. The condition is occasionally seen in very young children; however, the prevalence of bacterial vaginosis in this age group has not been reported.

(c) Group A and Group B streptococci

(d) *Escherichia coli*

(e) *Haemophilus influenzae*

Although the above three groups of organisms have been reported to cause vulvovaginitis, asymptomatic carriage may also occur. Positive bacterial culture from a vaginal swab may therefore not always signify pathogenicity. A true pathogenic role may be assumed if symptoms resolve with antibiotic treatment.

(d) *Chlamydia*

The prepubertal vagina is susceptible to chlamydial infection. This is in contrast to the adult where the cervix and urethra are the prime sites of infection. Prepubertal chlamydial infection should raise a strong suspicion of sexual abuse, although in the very young infection may have occurred by vertical transmission from the mother at birth. This may persist for up to 2 years after birth and possibly longer. Asymptomatic vaginal and rectal infection has been reported in as many as 15% of infants born to infected mothers. Conjunctivitis and pneumonitis are more common complications and have been reported in 50–70% of exposed infants.

(e) Gonorrhoea

This is a sexually transmitted infection and should be considered diagnostic of sexual abuse in the majority of cases.

2. Foreign bodies

Young girls occasionally insert small objects or pieces of toilet paper into the vagina as part of normal exploratory behaviour. With time these objects may give rise to a malodorous discharge. Insertion of objects that mimic a penis suggests possible sexual abuse rather than self-stimulation.

GENITAL IRRITATION

Vaginal discharge

This may cause vulval erythema and irritation secondary to persistent dampness. Alternatively vulval symptoms may be directly attributable to the initiating infection, e.g. *Candida*.

Threadworms

Generally considered a cause of anal irritation, threadworms may track to the vulval area and give rise to predominantly genital symptoms. Vulval erythema may be present.

Chemical irritants

'Bubble-bath', scented soaps and shampoos may cause an irritant dermatitis or a true contact dermatitis. As for adults, aqueous cream is a useful soap substitute.

Poor hygiene

Whereas excessive washing with scented soaps may cause problems, inadequate genital bathing and poor hygiene leading to prolonged exposure to urine or faeces may also predispose to irritation. Non-cotton and tight fitting underwear may aggravate symptoms.

Masturbation

Children masturbate or play with their genitalia from the time their hands can reach that far. This is considered a normal part of sexual development although it frequently generates a degree of anxiety in the parents. Public and 'excessive' masturbation may be seen in the learning disabled as part of their disability. The possibility of sexual abuse should be considered in other children, particularly if masturbation is performed in public.

Lichen sclerosus et atrophicus

This condition may affect young children and, to the unwary, may be misdiagnosed as evidence of sexual abuse. The clinical features are the same as seen in the adult.

Boys

Balanoposthitis is not an uncommon problem in uncircumcised young boys. Symptoms are usually mild and settle with simple measures, such as bathing. Recurrent inflammation is unusual and often associated with a non-retractile foreskin or poor hygiene. At birth the prepuce adheres to the glans penis in most infants. By 6 months 15% of infants have a retractile foreskin and by the age of 5 years just over 90% of boys can fully retract the foreskin. This increases to 99% by the age of 17 years. A inability to retract the foreskin may be due to phimosis which is a pathological scarring of the foreskin, often secondary to lichen sclerosus et atrophicus (balanitis xerotica obliterans). Phimosis should be distinguished from a normal but non-retractile foreskin. Preputial adhesions represent a stage in the normal process of separation of the two epithelial surfaces of the glans and the prepuce and will usually spontaneously resolve without treatment.

FURTHER READING

Holmes KK, Mardh P-A, Sparling PF *et al.* (eds). (1990). *Sexually Transmitted Diseases*. McGraw-Hill, New York.

Oates JK, Csonka G (eds) (1991). *Sexually Transmitted Diseases: A Textbook of Genitourinary Medicine*. WB Saunders, London.

Johnson AM, Wadsworth J, Wellings K *et al.* (1994). *Sexual Attitudes and Lifestyles*. Blackwell Scientific Publications, Oxford.

Mindel A (1989). *Herpes Simplex Virus*. Springer, Berlin.

Mindel A (ed.) (1994). *Genital Warts and Human Papillomavirus Infection*. Edward Arnold, London.

Ridley CM (ed.) (1988). *The Vulva*. Churchill Livingstone, London.

Ridley CM, Oriel JD, Robinson AJ (eds) (1992). *A Colour Atlas of Diseases of the Vulva*. Chapman and Hall Medical, London.

Singer A, Monaghan JM (1994). *Lower Genital Tract Precancer*. Blackwell Scientific Publications, Oxford.

Adler MW (ed.) (1991). *ABC of AIDS*. British Medical Journal Publications, London.

INDEX

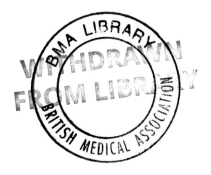